OTITIS MEDIA: COPING WITH THE EFFECTS IN THE CLASSROOM

Dorinne S. Davis, MA, CCC-A

HEAR YOU ARE, Inc.
Stanhope, New Jersey

Otitis Media: Coping with the Effects in the Classsroom

ISBN 0-9622326-0-2

DEDICATION

This book is dedicated to my wonderful family who lovingly supported me in my quest of assisting the child affected by otitis media: Warren, my husband, who encouraged me to meet my goal; Larissa, my daughter, who always gave me an extra hand; and Peter, my son, whose personal experiences with otitis media made me realize the depth of the problem.

FOREWORD

Serous, otitis media, middle ear effusion or ear infection, regardless of the label of choice, has become an issue of growing concern over the past 20 years. This concern is not without justification. Children with otitis media constitute the largest population of pediatric physician office visits each year. The literature boasts a wealth of opinions and studies hypothesizing and examining the possible relationship of recurrent and/or persistent otitis media and various areas of communication, listening and learning. Both parents and professionals are seeking answers to the question of what should be done to assist these children at home and in school.

The facts are that a considerable number of children have recurrent and/or persistent serous otitis media that begins in infancy, and that there is a high probability that these children are having some difficulty in communication, listening and/or learning. These difficulties may be manifest during the preschool years or they may be more subtle and go unnoticed until the child is faced with tasks required in the curriculum of formal education.

No classroom teacher providing educational services to school aged children escapes the presence of a child with current involvement with or history of recurrent and/or persistent serous otitis media. Large numbers of these children are receiving their educational instruction and experiences primarily in the regular public school classroom. Enhancement of the auditory environment, modifications in teaching strategies and adaptations in curriculum can provide a substantial benefit to children with recurrent and/or persistent otitis media and those who are bearing the residual effects of earlier involvement.

It would therefore seem that a logical move would be the development of a corpus of information that a classroom teacher could readily call upon to assist in his/her own understanding of the needs of otitis prone children and to provide suggestions for optimizing their educational experiences. This text by Dorinne Davis accomplishes this goal. It is a curriculum adaptation that can be a valuable aid to the classroom teacher. The goal is to enhance the classroom environment in order to augment learning for children who are affected by recurrent and/or persistent serous otitis media.

In this timely and valuable handbook, Ms. Davis presents information that is pertinent and reflective of current literature addressing otitis media in children. She also discusses behaviors of children who are actively experiencing middle ear effusion and those with histories of recurrent middle ear infections. Finally, she suggests and illustrates ways in which the learning environment can be adjusted or modified to provide benefit to these children.

M. Suzanne Hasenstab, Ph.D.
Associate Professor
Assistant Director: Audiology/Speech Pathology
Medical College of Virginia

TABLE OF CONTENTS

IV. SOCIALIZATION

PREFACE

Background

Otitis Media, or middle ear infection, is a major health problem for young children which can cause them serious learning problems. These problems are often subtle in nature. They may not be recognized as problems until children meet failure in the later elementary grades. Teachers, if they understand the causes and possible methods of intervention, can prevent or lessen this failure.

As an audiologist who has specialized in the educational management of children with hearing impairments, I have had the opportunity to work with children with varying degrees of hearing difficulty. A significant emphasis of my work has been with the child who has had a history of middle ear infections. Identifying and assisting these children at risk is paramount for their success. The classroom teacher has the initial contact with the children and should be knowledgeable in the effects otitis media has on the children's learning.

I developed this curriculum adaptation first as a way to alert classroom teachers to the special areas of weakness generally associated with these children. Then, I have tried to provide the kind of activities and ideas that can be used by teachers in their regular classroom situations with their regular curriculum to assist these students to develop appropriate language skills. Next, I provide forms that proved useful in the Kinnelon, New Jersey School System. Lastly, I have included an extensive bibliography which will allow for further reading.

Purpose

This curriculum adaptation is designed to:

1. Provide a methodology that will enable the classroom teacher to recognize the needs of the otitis media affected child in the classroom.

2. Discuss areas of concern related to otitis media.

3. Suggest activities that can enhance these children's learning in the classroom situation.

4. Show ways to enhance the learning environment by considering the acoustics, using small classroom settings or using sound field amplification in large classroom settings.

An individualized therapy plan administered by a specialist may be best for an individual child. But that therapy will be most effective when the classroom teacher provides reinforcing activities. And unfortunately, some children with subtle needs are overlooked. Providing an easy way to use methodology may help teachers to identify and assist these children at an earlier age.

Perhaps this curriculum adaptation will help classroom teachers to become more knowledgeable about the needs of this population. Many of the techniques presented are already being used by many fine teachers, but perhaps not in conjunction with other activities as presented here. Helping the world of otitis media affected children to become more meaningful may be just the boost these children need to become more productive members of society.

Audience

This guide was written for regular classroom teachers. They are very often the first to see the children who have suffered with otitis media. They may be unaware of the importance of assisting this population as early as possible. Teachers in other specialty fields may also find the information helpful in understanding the overall developmental needs of otitis media affected children.

Author's Assumption

Although language is the basis for communication, this curriculum adaptation will not try to "teach" language per se. That will be left to the Speech/Language Pathologists. The author does recognize that in-depth analysis of the child's language and communication skills is important to the total performance of the otitis media child. In this curriculum adaptation, problem areas associated with the otitis media child are incorporated into an adaptive curriculum based on a strong language-based program. Some of the skills taught include language activities, but are not meant to teach to any one particular language deficit. Even though the ideal time for assisting a child is during any episode from infancy onward, this curriculum is adapted for use with children from age three and older since those are the children that the author services at present.

The author assumes that any program will utilize the Speech/ Language Pathologist to evaluate an individual child's specific language problem areas.

Most language screening tests are not sensitive to the specific areas of concern related to the otitis media affected child. Dr. M. Suzanne Hasenstab, in her book *Language Learning and Otitis Media*, presents an excellent evaluative and habilitative discussion on language for the child with recurrent otitis media. She also states that children affected by recurrent otitis media need to be guided to take "knowledge that they possess (language content), what they already know about communication (language form), and use it appropriately."

She further states that the two paramount issues regarding learners are:

• children must be able to respond to different tasks with different strategies

• children may arrive at the same result from different perspectives or approaches.

This must be considered within the confines of a structured curriculum. Provision must be made that will allow for alternate modes of intake and response.

Acknowledgements

A special thanks to:

• Mrs. Patricia Hills of the Kinnelon Public Library for locating numerous research papers necessary for the background of this publication

• E. Patricia Birsner, my editor, for her invaluable contribution of knowledge and organization

• Friends, family and colleagues for their continuous support.

• Kathy Teasley, my typesetter, for never complaining about all the changes I had to make.

INTRODUCTION

Almost all classroom teachers are familiar with the term "middle ear infection." But the educational significance of that term may be something to which they give no more than a passing thought. They know that they may need to give children who have had a number of middle ear infections preferential seating. But unless an educational audiologist is on the staff, often little is done to ensure the appropriateness of the "preferential seating," let alone proper educational management.

"Middle ear infection" is the lay terminology for otitis media. It is defined as an inflammation of the middle ear. Otitis media can be further delineated as to whether fluid is present and what kind of fluid it is, the length of its onset and its duration, and its frequency. Medical people often attach such terms as serous (type of fluid), recurrent (frequently recurring), acute (less than three weeks, a quick onset with pain/fever), chronic (longer than three weeks, repeated attacks, and possible perforation of the eardrum), suppurative (pus present), and purulent (pus filled) to their diagnoses and their discussions to provide information about the seriousness of otitis media in a particular child.[1]

Otitis media is one of the most common infectious childhood diseases. Doctors estimate that between 75 and 95 percent of all children experience at least one middle ear infection before entering school. (Hasenstab, 1987) The term 'otitis prone' is applied to children who experience six or more episodes of otitis media before they reach the age of six. (Howie, Ploussard and Sloyer, 1975) Otitis media can lead either to a temporary conductive hearing loss or to sensorineural loss which is permanent. The ratio between these two types of loss in pre-school populations is from 11 to 1 to 18 to 1, depending upon age factors. (Brooks, 1979) The loss is more pronounced especially when the onset of the first episode is in the child's first year of life. (Northern and Downs, 1984)

Children learn language during their first few years of life. If they are to acquire language, their auditory systems need to receive consistent auditory input from their environment. They learn language through an established auditory feedback system.

An auditory feedback system involves the use of an auditory memory retrieval system whereby a listener compares any insufficient incoming messages with past experiences. If a child has received inconsistent input for whatever reason, the retrieval system has difficulty operating because it does not have enough consistent events stored from which to piece together a conclusion. Therefore, the child can make an incorrect judgment about what he or she heard.

---

[1] Further detailed information about the types of otitis media can be found in Hasenstab, *Language Learning and Otitis Media*, 1987, and Kavanaugh, *Otitis Media and Child Development*, 1986.

Note that school age children do not have to be currently experiencing middle ear infections to be at risk. Prior episodes of otitis media, especially in the first year or two of life, can result in later problems. Children automatically base and make their decisions on prior information. If they received inconsistent or deficient input of the auditory signal, the information will be received incorrectly, and the store of information upon which they build future references will be inaccurate. Thus, they are more likely to make incorrect assumptions and give wrong answers. This failure can diminish their self esteem over time. Children are like everyone else — they don't like to make errors when the task at hand precludes failure. So, they may react with a number of unsatisfactory behaviors — they may be overactive, lack attention, use other senses, cling to parent figures, etc.

POSSIBLE PROBLEM AREAS FOR
THE OTITIS MEDIA AFFECTED CHILD

Children must have consistent auditory input for the proper development of their audition, cognition, language and socialization skills.

Audition

Audition is the ability to receive auditory input and make use of it appropriately, receiving the stimulus and recognizing that it is music, words, noise or other sound. For otitis media affected children, special attention must be paid to the auditory and listening environment since they may have difficulty listening and attending in the presence of extraneous noise or poor acoustical environments. They may be unable to hear and separate out the individual sounds of letters, to blend words together, or to follow through with verbal directions. They often have a short attention span. They do not "use" sound appropriately and tend to ignore auditory stimuli. They may say "huh" or "what" or have slow, delayed responses to sound. The sounds they do receive may not organize into anything that is meaningful to them. As a result, they may be slow task starters and fail to complete assigned tasks.

For children with deficits in audition, learning to attend to sounds, to "listen" is extremely important. They must learn to pay attention, to try to sort out the various sounds. Placing them in environments with good acoustics, in quiet areas without distracting noise, or in situations where sound is amplified on headsets or through assistive listening systems can help them learn this important skill.

Verbal social interaction is important in communication. The listener must attend, and then respond appropriately. The speaker must discern whether the listener has comprehended. But the breakdown can be in the context – or in the condition of either the listener or the speaker. If the speaker speaks too rapidly, too softly, mumbles, doesn't enunciate clearly, or turns away from the listener, the child cannot "hear" or process the sound correctly – and that breakdown is caused by the speaker. Unsuccessful attempts at communication, either initiated by the child or requiring a response can result in frustration, poor self concept, a sense of failure, and resulting inappropriate behavior.

Listening must be meaningful. Skill area mastery itself is not essential at first. But utilizing the skill areas within meaningful contexts is beneficial. Listening goes beyond hearing acuity and relates the incoming message to the message base in the brain. This message base provides a composite of previous input from which to draw outcomes for the present input.

Cognition

Cognition is the knowledge base of learning. Children's cognition is drawn from stored sensory information which allows them to make sense of their environment. Cognition helps them to organize, categorize, restructure and store information for future use. It requires that they develop learning strategies that will enhance and increase their knowledge base and help them to apply that knowledge in meaningful ways.

Otitis media affected children have varying degrees of auditory deficits, so are forced to rely on their other senses to learn. They may require extra processing time. They may say "what" or "huh" to buy that extra time. They function best in a small, orderly, familiar world, and may look at you with blank confused faces when faced with something new and unfamiliar. They may have difficulty recalling names, talk around or circumlocute an item instead of naming it, have difficulty answering even simple questions, and frequently have difficulty with spelling because they have difficulty with the sounds that make up the words.

One of the problems of otitis media in educational terms is the difficulty of knowing what element is being misrepresented at what time in an individual child's development. The degree of hearing loss and the fluctuation of the condition create inconsistent and altered stimuli for the child to hear and process. As all children grow and mature differently, it becomes especially difficult to determine what is happening to an individual child. Each case appears to be unique. However, general areas of difficulty can be identified, although an individual child will not have all the academic and social behaviors that can be associated with otitis media. Yet even those children who do not exhibit a particular deficit still benefit from the learning and teaching modes that are different from the standard.

Language Skills

When children develop language or linguistic skills, they internalize the rules of communication so that spontaneous verbal interactions can occur. For otitis media affected children, this internalization may be incomplete. As a result, their conversations may jump back and forth through different topics within one conversation.

They may have difficulty recalling exactly the right word; have difficulty waiting for their turn to speak; may use a rehearsed phrase to mean many things — for example, too big to mean large, big, many, etc.; may have difficulty with plurals, possessives and irregular past tenses; be unable to predict story outcomes; and may be very literal and unable to draw conclusions and understand inferences.

Although research methodologies and definitions differ, the literature generally agrees that otitis prone children do have academic difficulties. The performance area deficits have been linked to word recognition, reading, spelling and computational arithmetic. Freeman and Parkins (1979) report that reading disorders are 15 times greater in otitis media affected children versus children with no history of otitis media.

The author believes that even though the literature has not been definitive in agreeing about problems associated with otitis media, functioning children who have histories of otitis media or who have otitis media at present can benefit from adaptive input modes of learning. The result will be better functioning students with higher self esteem. Some school districts allow children to progress through the mainstream until actual failure can be documented – usually around grade three or four. By this time, it may be too late, and children's low self-esteem patterns are set for life. As educators, we should be concerned that all of the outcomes of students' learning are positive. Varying our teaching modes may be necessary if we are to reach this goal.

Unfortunately, many school districts are not servicing otitis media affected children appropriately. The children are not being identified early enough or are not being sufficiently helped. Time constraints may not allow for the speech/language pathologist to develop the in-depth language profile that is so important. This curriculum adaptation can provide teachers with ways in which they can assist all children, whether or not they are in a regular classroom.

Of course, all children with recurrent otitis media are not exactly alike and they all do not require the same intervention structure. Their individual language needs are different. Therefore, a "cookbook" approach or so-called "therapeutic programming" will not be helpful, given the differences in the otitis media population. This curriculum adaptation is designed to help the classroom teacher first to become aware of the problems of otitis media affected children, then to learn how to make the necessary allowances or changes to meet their needs. Some of the suggestions incorporate language activities.

Socialization

Social development is also an area of concern with otitis media affected children. Cantwell and Baker, in 1977 and again in 1980, suggested that children with receptive deficits show a greater degree of inappropriateness in the social and behavior categories than do children without those deficits. Auditory-based language problems, such as those associated with otitis media, are deficits in input and reception that occur because of interference with the reception of auditory information. In a study by Beratis, et al (1979), an infant with an intermittent hearing loss secondary to otitis media was observed. Unless the child was able to maintain visual contact with someone during periods of decreased hearing, crying and restlessness were noted. But when the child's hearing returned to normal, so did the behavior.

In pre-school and elementary school children, the social behaviors that have been associated with histories of otitis media are distractibility, overactivity, social withdrawal, inattention, and inappropriate response behaviors. Teachers often judge these as immature behaviors, but perhaps a reason is behind that immaturity. The label "self-centered" or "spoiled" may be applied when in reality, the children's inability to process the environment has forced them to try to bring order to their world in the only way they know. They need to order their own world first before they can behave "maturely." They don't have the skills to reach beyond what is frustrating them.

An important part of any successful program for this population is to include the children's parents in the learning process. They must be made aware of their children's needs and frustrations, and be given ways to enhance communication at home. Consistent carryover is important if the children are going to develop appropriately.

More importantly, the total child must be considered and his or her needs met. With knowledgeable teachers, perhaps many of the "failures" can be avoided. This adaptation is only a beginning – a guide to begin enhancing the otitis media affected child's total education. As you begin to apply some of the basic principals to your teaching, you will find many ways to include specific techniques and emphasize other areas of importance based upon your own school curriculum. You can add more areas or delete those which don't seem appropriate to your individual school.

CURRICULUM OVERVIEW

Goals

To create an awareness in classroom teachers of the difficulty the otitis media affected child may have in learning and developing.

To provide various ways the classroom teacher can assist the otitis media affected child that will enhance learning and foster positive self-esteem.

Objectives

Audition
To understand the auditory difficulties related to the otitis media affected child and learn various strategies to enable the child to overcome those difficulties.

Cognition
To understand the cognitive related difficulties related to the otitis media affected child and develop the ability to use a variety of strategies to overcome those deficits.

Language Skills
To understand the linguistic related difficulties related to the otitis media affected child and employ a variety of strategies to assist the child to overcome those difficulties.

Socialization
To understand the social inadequacies that the otitis media affected child may have and learn to use strategies to help the child overcome those inadequacies.

Arrangement of Assistance

Possible problem areas are listed in relationship to each objective.

Techniques for curriculum adaptation are given for each problem area.

Extra information, materials, and/or references are provided.

Problem Areas

I. Audition

1.1 The child has difficulty attending or listening in the presence of background noise.

1.2 The child has difficulty hearing the individual sounds of letters.

1.3 The child has difficulty blending sounds into words.

1.4 The child has difficulty following through with verbal directions.

1.5 The child does not "use" sound appropriately (also child tends to ignore sound).

1.6 The child says "huh" or "what" frequently.

1.7 The child has a short attention span.

1.8 The child appears to have a delayed response to sound.

1.9 The child is a slow task starter.

1.10 The child fails to complete assigned tasks.

1.11 The child has difficulty hearing differences between sounds or phonemes.

1.12 The child has difficulty understanding and repeating words of many syllables or sounds. Common error words are: spaghetti/pasghetti and animal/aminal/amimal.

II. Cognition

2.1 The child learns better through senses other than auditory.

2.2 The child says "huh" or "what" frequently.

2.3 The child needs extra processing time.

2.4 The child functions best in his/her own orderly world.

2.5 The child looks at you with blank confused face.

2.6 The child has difficulty with name recall.

2.7 The child talks around an item or circumlocutes the item instead of giving the vocabulary word.

2.8 The child has difficulty with simple questions.

2.9 The child has difficulty with spelling.

2.10 The child has difficulty with mental arithmetic.

2.11 The child has difficulty with reading. (This area is deliberately kept broad, although it could be broken down into sound blending, context clues, etc. For more in-depth ideas, consult a reading specialist, but make sure he/she understands the intricacies of otitis media histories.)

III. Language Skills

3.1 The child has difficulty recalling the name of an item; will describe it or talk around it, but will not recall the name.

3.2 The child has difficulties with word relationships such as spatial, temporal, or cause and effect.

3.3 The child's conversations jump through different topics within one conversation.

3.4 The child answers questions inappropriately.

3.5 The child has difficulty waiting for his/her turn.

3.6 The child may use a rehearsed phrase to mean many things. ("too big" may mean "too large," "too many," etc.)

3.7 The child has difficulty predicting story outcomes.

3.8 The child has difficulty with plurals, possessives, and irregular past tenses.

3.9 The child is very literal.

3.10 The child uses inappropriate pronoun references. Example: may start with one form and then change the form later.

3.11 The child has difficulty extracting the main idea of a paragraph or story.

3.12 The child has difficulty putting his/her thoughts into words.

IV. Socialization

4.1 Child exhibits overactivity: he/she uses it as a means of investigation, goal fulfillment or a method of communication. The actions are often purposeful.

4.2 The child is distractible: other senses interfere with the ability to concentrate on a task.

4.3 The child does not participate in class, but when he/she does, may give an inappropriate response.

4.4 The child manipulates objects or uses class materials inappropriately (bangs pencil on the desk, stares at a pencil on the desk while the teacher is talking, places body physically away from the teacher, such as turning sideways on the chair).

4.5 The child is prone to tantrums.

4.6 The child withdraws from classroom activity (also includes the category of daydreaming).

4.7 The child prefers to be alone or removed when the noise levels get too much.

4.8 The child likes to be read to.

4.9 The child is often unaware of the needs of others (also the intentions of others).

4.10 The child is often considered "immature."

4.11 The child has difficulty taking turns.

4.12 The child can't wait to say what his/her thoughts are (also applies to the child who simply shouts out answers).

4.13 The child prefers the company of younger children or adults.

CURRICULUM ADAPTATIONS AND ACTIVITIES

Objective Information

The need for the objectives and subobjectives as stated will vary with the skills of the child. At first glance, otitis media affected children may appear to have excellent language, speech and academic skills. But surprising gaps may be evidenced as they progress through school. All of the children with otitis media will not experience all the problem areas presented but may benefit from the special attention the adaptions provide anyway. Therefore, meeting children's overall educational needs at an early age is important. The earlier help is started, the greater the degree of success, and the less likely an individual child will develop a negative attitude and low self-esteem.

The curriculum adaptation is written on a combination psychosocial-auralinguistic basis. The total child is considered, not just certain portions of his or her development. Specific skill mastery is not stressed. Understanding the child and adapting teaching methods to suit the otitis media affected child's needs is more important. Although the four main areas of audition, cognition, language skills and socialization are included, each area overlaps the others and they all are interrelated. The approach is a global one – teaching to specific language skills is not included because these skills need to be individualized for each child by a specialist.

Maintaining appropriate auditory input is stressed throughout to avoid future difficulties. Since amplification has been demonstrated as a means to provide sufficient continuous auditory input, one method suggested is sound field amplification. To use this method, the teacher wears a wireless microphone and his or her voice is amplified over the entire classroom at 10-15 decibels above normal conversational speech. This technique has been shown to increase the scores of all children on the California Achievement Test (CAT) in the fourth grade, but the increase is especially significant for those children with histories of otitis media. (Ray, et. al, 1984) In the Kinnelon, New Jersey schools, where many of the children in the Pre-School Handicapped classroom have histories of otitis media, this method is being used extensively. (Lovas, 1985) Personal sound amplifiers are being used as well for children experiencing otitis media episodes in the Kinnelon Schools through a loaner bank system. (Davis, 1988) The device is put on a child during periods of decreased hearing. The program is monitored by the educational audiologist.

In the activity section, the general problems are stated. Techniques for curriculum adaptations are presented next, followed by additional information, materials, and/or references. One aid that will be mentioned frequently is a technique the author labels as having your "eyes help your ears." This will be mentioned throughout. In this technique, the teacher asks the children to use another of their senses, in this case, the eyes, to supplement their hearing. Whenever possible, the children look at objects, colors, etc., when they are mentioned to assist in memory recall. The

11

children may also be asked to visualize the response in their heads. For example, if they are asked to "circle the dog," they can visualize the circle in their mind before actually following through with the direction. All of the techniques suggested have been helpful with individual children. Try different techniques with different children to find out which approaches work best.

Four major adaptations will be stressed as important to the overall success of these children: sound field amplification, personal sound amplifiers, good classroom acoustics, and a smaller number of children in the classroom or working group. Any or all of these may not be available to the teacher, but this does not diminish their importance.

Techniques for Curriculum Adaptation	Extra Information, Materials or References

1.1   The child has difficulty attending or listening in the presence of background noise.

1.1.a   Minimize extraneous noise by treating the room with sound absorbing materials. Rugs or carpeting can be used in areas where group activity takes place. Curtains on windows can absorb sound. Book shelves placed strategically can absorb sound.

                                     1.1.a.1   Carpeting or rugs can be obtained in fairly decent shape from parents who are having new carpeting installed.

                                     1.1.a.2   For further sources on classroom acoustics, see Berg, (1987); Ross, (1972)

1.1.b   Minimize classroom interruptions as much as possible. When the child is doing seat work, limit discussions with other staff members to outside of the classroom. If child is doing seat work and another group is working in the room, place the child as far away from the group as possible.

1.1.c   When the child is doing seat work, ear muffs or ear plugs may be used to block out extraneous noise.

1.1.d   Sound field amplification amplifies the teacher's voice and may override the background noise sufficiently for the child to attend.

                                     1.1.d.1   See appendix for sources.

1.1.e   When teaching, remain stationary. Moving around the room creates a visual disturbance as well as an auditory disturbance (the sound of the voice changes with the teacher's position) and breaks the child's concentration for attending.

AUDITION

Techniques for Curriculum Adaptation	Extra Information, Materials or References

1.1 **The child has difficulty attending or listening in the presence of background noise.** (Continued)

1.1.f   Give additional input. Restate, rephrase, restructure the teaching message so that a variety of input may be processed.

1.1.f.1   Children will tire easily after having to attend for long periods. Allow for frequent breaks in between demanding lessons. Young children, even in grades one or two, need actual play time to diminish the stress of attending or listening.

1.1.g   Speak clearly and slowly. Background noise can mask or alter how speech sounds are heard. Rapid speech is difficult for the child to perceive with the added interference of noise.

1.1.h   Speak directly to the child's face if possible. Position the child so that he/she is in front of you. When the head is turned, the volume of the voice is lowered. The child needs constant direct input of sound whenever possible.

1.1.i   Request verbal feedback periodically. This helps pinpoint misinterpretations and also encourages the child to listen. If the child heard incorrectly, simply restate and rephrase what was said.

1.1.j   Use gestures to point to discussion objects but don't allow body language/ gestures to override the verbal content. These gestures can act as a visual disturbance.

1.1.k   Repeat directions to child individually whenever appropriate.

Techniques for Curriculum Adaptation	Extra Information, Materials or References

1.1 **The child has difficulty attending or listening in the presence of background noise.** (Continued)

1.1.l A visual aid such as an overhead projector can visually assist in directing the child's input to the task. It also can be used for summation.

1.1.l.1 For some children, this may take away necessary facial input messages which the child relies on for comprehension. If using the overhead, make sure the room is light enough for the child to see the teacher's face. The teacher should still face the child.

1.1.m Have the child utilize other senses for reinforcement. For example: "use the eyes to help the ears" when appropriate. This may target the focus away from the noise. Watch for misinterpretation of words due to noise blocking sound.

1.1.m.1 Technique discussed in Objective Information.

1.1.n Personal Sound Amplification may be used in small group instruction or one-on-one instruction where the amplifier can be placed close to the teacher's voice. The child is receiving the teacher's voice directly over the noise of the classroom, although the classroom noise is also amplified. The teacher's voice in relation to the background noise is greater. This is referred to as the Signal to Noise Ratio or S/N.

1.1.n.1 This can be accomplished relatively inexpensively. Various makes of units and a source for the units is in the appendix.

1.1.n.2 This system should generally not be used all the time because it can amplify all the classroom noise which may be too much for the child.

1.1.n.3 Care should be taken not to overamplify the child. The setting should be minimal. Ideally, the system should be controlled by the educational audiologist.

AUDITION

Techniques for Curriculum Adaptation	Extra Information, Materials or References

1.1 **The child has difficulty attending or listening in the presence of background noise.** (Continued)

1.1.o A Sound Enhancement System is another way to get direct auditory input of the teacher's voice. The S/N ratio allows the teacher's voice to be heard directly over the classroom noise.

1.1.o.1 Many companies are coming out with this sort of system. Different units and sources are listed in the appendix.

1.1.o.2 With this kind of system, both the teacher and the child wear a part of the system. It amplifies sound and eliminates the extraneous sound. The microphone can be passed around so that other participants can be heard by the child, as well.

1.2 **The child has difficulty hearing the individual sounds of letters.**

1.2.a Find additional clues to emphasize phonics. Some reading systems utilize a specified sound per sound combination with a set picture and name per sound card. This system can be helpful in getting the child, through rote repetition, to associate sound and letter.

1.2.a.1 *Open Court Reading System* by Open Court Publication Co., Il, is one such system.

1.2.b It is helpful to teach whole word units rather than emphasize hearing the individual sound which is extremely difficult for this child.

1.2.b.1 (Dobie & Berlin, 1979.) For the otitis media affected child, reading skills developed more rapidly when complete sentences were taught rather than words in isolation. Therefore, reading is frequently better served by teaching whole words and sentence units versus blending and sounding out words.

Techniques for Curriculum Adaptation	Extra Information, Materials or References

1.2   The child has difficulty hearing the individual sounds of letters. (Continued)

	1.2.b.2 The child may have difficulty hearing and distinguishing low intensity words such as a, an, the, on, up, etc. This may interfere with his/her ability to hear and remember the sounds within these words.
	1.2.b.3 General rules of thumb with isolated speech sounds are: 1) low pitched sounds are easier to hear than high pitched sounds, 2) vowels are easier to hear than consonants and 3) voiced consonants are easier to hear than unvoiced consonants. However, when combined in words, any of these rules may change due to the duration of the sound, how it is used in combination with other sounds, its placement in a sentence, the intonation, rhythm pattern of speech and rate of speech.
	1.2.b.4 The child may have difficulty hearing pitch, loudness, rhythm, duration or timbre of sounds and therefore, may not be able to distinguish the individual sounds within words.
1.2.c Word association is another way to teach the word units.	
1.2.d Stress reading and writing together. Language experience stories allow the child to use his/her own language and read back the message unit.	1.2.d.1 The teacher can write down the story as the child relates it. The child can then read it back.
1.2.e Use sound field amplification to amplify the teacher's voice so that the child will hear the sounds better.	

AUDITION

Techniques for Curriculum Adaptation	Extra Information, Materials or References
1.2 **The child has difficulty hearing the individual sounds of letters.** (Continued)	
1.2.f Make sure the acoustics of the teaching area are not creating additional sound cues such as reverberation of the sounds, thereby creating more confusion in the listening situation.	1.2.f.1 Refer to 1.1.a
1.2.g Ensure the child is away from extraneous noise when teaching verbally the sounds of letters.	
1.2.h Emphasize visual coding and decoding of words directly to meaning and avoid the teaching of individual sounds at first.	
1.2.i Utilize a sing-song approach to learning the sounds of letters. Utilizing another input mode may be beneficial for some.	
1.2.j The child may hear sounds in isolation but not when extraneous noise is present. Introduce sound in quiet and gradually present noise over time. Make sure adequate time has been given to hear, associate and learn sound first.	
1.2.k Personal sound amplification can be utilized when teaching the individual sounds of words. The increased intensity of the auditory input can stimulate how the sound is perceived. Over time, this extra input can make retention of the letter sounds easier for some children.	1.2.k.1 See 1.1.n

Techniques for Curriculum Adaptation	Extra Information, Materials or References

1.2   The child has difficulty hearing the individual sounds of letters. (Continued)

1.2.1   A sound enhancement system may also be beneficial for the child to receive and perceive the sound of the letter.

1.2.1.1   See 1.1.o

1.2.m   Tape the sounds of letters on a tape recorder in random order or in a set teaching order. Using a ditto sheet with corresponding sounds as well as different sounds, have the child pick out the letters having the same sounds used on the tape.

1.2m.1   Allow the child to rehearse the sounds by himself/herself. Set up a self-check method, so the child can monitor his/her own skills and not feel a low self esteem when one is missed.

1.3   The child has difficulty blending sounds into words.

1.3.a   Try to avoid adding spacing between the sounds of words being blended.

1.3.a.1   The child may be able to hear the individual sounds of letters but when someone attempts to blend these sounds into a word such as 's_a_t', the space between the sounds actually changes how the sounds are made and heard versus how the sounds are made and heard within a word as a whole. There are subtle differences in the pitch, loudness, rhythm, duration, and timbre of each sound. The otitis media affected child who has struggled to learn the word as a whole when learning language and may have heard it inconsistently, can have an even greater difficulty if the sounds are altered within the word which he/she is attempting to read in parts.

AUDITION

Techniques for Curriculum Adaptation	Extra Information, Materials or References

1.3   The child has difficulty blending sounds into words. (Continued)

	1.3.a.2 The child may simply have difficulty sequencing the separated sounds. The connection of the sounds into the whole word may have more meaning.
1.3.b Try blending the sounds together within the word but at a faster rate.	1.3.b.1 The closer one can come to approximating the word in its entirety, the more likely the child will comprehend what the word is.
1.3.c Try a whole word reading approach versus a blending technique.	1.3.c.1 As children with otitis media histories tend to have difficulties comprehending the individual sounds of letters, they sometimes have difficulty understanding an altered word resulting from a blending separation. The whole word approach may be more helpful because it uses the word as a basic unit of reference. The children may know what a whole word sounds like and they need to learn what it looks like.
	1.3.c.2 Word families as whole words can be taught teaching the same individual concepts. For example, the long 'a_e' can be taught by giving the missing consonant for as many words as the children can come up with. Afterwards, the 'a_e' can be discussed. Encourage the children to provide input from their own reference points – the words they know. Then have them identify the similarities in the words that you want to teach. This idea can be adapted for any basic reading skill being taught.

Techniques for Curriculum Adaptation	Extra Information, Materials or References

1.3   The child has difficulty blending sounds into words. (Continued)

1.3.d Try using personal sound amplification between teacher and child.	1.3.d.1 By providing a slightly louder input, the child may be able to compensate for the changes of the sounds within the word that are altered by duration and rhythm. If the child is significantly bothered by the time change between the sounds, this may not be helpful. However, the idea has been effective in many cases for the author.
1.3.e Try raising the intensity of your voice when saying each sound, in particular the softer speech sounds.	1.3.e.1 Otitis media affected children often have difficulty with low intensity words and low intensity sounds. Some of the low intensity sounds are: t, p, ch, s, m, f and k.
	1.3.e.2 Unstressed phonemes are often missed. When separating out the sounds within words, emphasize each phoneme group (which is often individual sounds) versus each individual letter sound.
	1.3.e.3 Remember that low pitched sounds, such as vowels and voiced consonants (ex: b, d) are easier to hear. High pitched sounds, such as unvoiced consonants (ex: s, k, f) are harder to hear.
	1.3.e.4 Placement of a word within a sentence is important. It should be considered when determining whether a speech sound is difficult to hear. Placement will vary the stress of the word.
1.3.f Instead of blending each letter sound, try blending words by phonemes.	1.3.f.1 Very often the child can perceive phonemes in quiet or isolation.

AUDITION

Techniques for Curriculum Adaptation	Extra Information, Materials or References

1.3　**The child has difficulty blending sounds into words.** (Continued)

1.3.g　Ensure that the listening/teaching environment is fairly quiet.

1.3.g.1　See 1.3.f.1

1.3.g.2　Sound field amplification, personal sound amplifiers, or sound enhancement systems may be utilized during the reading lessons to ensure that the child has optimum listening capabilities. The child needs to be provided with as many ways to succeed as possible.

1.3.h　Try teaching the word in a cloze sentence technique.

1.3.h.1　The otitis media affected child has demonstrated that growth is more rapid for sentences (Dobie and Berlin, 1979). Provide him/her with the ingredients to succeed. If the child learns better through whole sentences versus words in isolation, then provide that opportunity. The cloze technique can allow him/her to draw from his/her linguistic knowledge to fit together any missing pieces. For example: John saw the red ___ drive away. The child can draw from the words 'drive,' 'red,' and 'saw' the clues to derive 'car'. Then given this prior knowledge, the new word 'car' or 'truck' might be introduced.

1.3.i　Provide as many visual or tactile reinforcements as possible to back up the production of the sounds.

1.3.i.1　The child can benefit from multisensory input. By providing numerous input modes, the child has more information from which to draw a response.

Techniques for Curriculum Adaptation	Extra Information, Materials or References

1.3   **The child has difficulty blending sounds into words.** (Continued)

1.3.j	Use word association techniques.	1.3.j.1	This can help the speed of remembering and retaining information. Whatever techniques of word association that have been successful in the past can be tried with the otitis media affected child.
1.3.k	Try having the child write the word as he/she is trying to blend it.	1.3.k.1	Extend this to writing and reading simultaneously. The multi-modalities reinforce each other.

1.4   **The child has difficulty following through with verbal directions.**

1.4.a	Have the child verbally repeat the direction.	1.4.a.1	The child may be able to repeat exactly what has been said when standing in front of the teacher, but forgets it on the way back to the desk. Sometimes, by allowing the child to quietly repeat the instructions verbally a number of times, he/she is able to draw upon memory skills to remember the direction.
		1.4.a.2	The child is having the message reinforced through auditory, verbal and tactile reinforcement. The combination of the verbal response (including the articulators) with the auditory has proven to be very successful.

AUDITION

Techniques for Curriculum Adaptation	Extra Information, Materials or References

1.4 **The child has difficulty following through with verbal directions.** (Continued)

1.4.b Encourage the child with goal directed activities.	1.4.b.1 Often the child can repeat the direction to the teacher but has difficulty starting the task. The child needs to be provided with directions for initiating, continuing and finishing a task. Sometimes, he or she simply needs a signal or clue which will provide an impetus for starting.
1.4.c Repeat the direction exactly as it was said the first time. Then rephrase it.	1.4.c.1 Frequently, the otitis media affected child is afraid to ask for clarification. He/she may not have understood the linguistic information. Rephrasing provides more input.
	1.4.c.2 Sometimes, the child has simply not heard enough of the message to comprehend it. By repeating it exactly as said, he/she has time to process the same information again. Rephrasing adds extra information.
1.4.d Encourage the child to ask for clarification no matter how silly it may seem.	1.4.d.1 Having the courage to ask for clarification will only develop over time. If the child has found that adults don't want to clarify when he/she is uncertain, the child may be reluctant to open up to a new person. Only through constant reinforcement and by feeling that he/she can be safe with you will the child want to try breaking through his/her own internal safety zone.

Techniques for Curriculum Adaptation	Extra Information, Materials or References

1.4   The child has difficulty following through with verbal directions. (Continued)

1.4.e	Be aware that some of the message may not be comprehended.	1.4.e.1	The child may not have understood the language of the direction. Provide the child with as many ways as possible for comprehension: rephrase, use visual cues, allow tactile input, etc.
		1.4.e.2	The child may not have heard all of the message or may have heard the message incorrectly. For example, the child may hear the word 'pat' for 'fat' and then the sentence, "mark the fat cat," would be confusing.
1.4.f	For the older child, allow him/her to write down the direction.	1.4.f.1	By writing the direction, another sense has been included and again, the child has been given more information to process the direction.
1.4.g	For the older child utilize a note taker.	1.4.g.1	A note taker is a way for one friend to write down the directions or homework assignments with a copy being given to the other student. If the child has to write down the direction, he/she often cannot do both: listen and write. Sometimes the act of writing down the message makes him/her forget the whole message. The child only understands the part that he or she has written. Note takers are ways for the child to listen and learn without missing some of the message.
1.4.h	Encourage the child to "use your eyes to help your ears."	1.4.h.1	See Objective Information on page 11.

AUDITION

Techniques for Curriculum Adaptation	Extra Information, Materials or References

1.4   **The child has difficulty following through with verbal directions.** (Continued)

1.4.i   Provide activities which can develop sequential memory skills.

     1.4.i.1   Verbal repetition can be helpful.

     1.4.i.2   Using the "eyes to help your ears" technique can be beneficial.

     1.4.i.3   Use organizational skill techniques for the child to monitor his/her own progress.

     1.4.i.4   Frequently with a complex direction, the child may remember and understand part of the task, but may not remember the second or third part of it; or may remember the last part and not remember the first or second part.

1.4.j   Make sure that the child is attending before starting the task.

     1.4.j.1   The child's attention may be elsewhere for the initial part of the direction. He/she may tune in by the middle but missed the beginning. The child may or may not be aware of this, and may not be able to ask for clarification.

     1.4.j.2   After giving the assignment, it can be helpful to summarize and restate the entire task again, in order.

1.4.k   Emphasize key words in the directional task by raising the intensity of the voice.

     1.4.k.1   The raised intensity brings extra awareness to the key words. The child is aware of the importance of those words because of the extra input which was given to them.

Techniques for Curriculum Adaptation	Extra Information, Materials or References

1.4   The child has difficulty following through with verbal directions. (Continued)

1.4.1   Ensure that the acoustic environment is appropriate.

1.4.1.1   Poor acoustical environments do not allow the child to perceive the directional tasks adequately. Consider all aspects of the environment: the classroom lighting, curtains, floor material, and open spaces.

1.4.1.2   When extraneous noise is a distraction, morphological markers, short words, and inflections can be missed. With directions, these words are often the ones that are important in giving meaning.

1.4.m   Sound field amplification, personal sound amplification and sound enhancement systems can provide the extra input necessary to process the direction.

1.4.n   Provide numerous vocabulary development experiences on directional words and word parts. Make sure that the vocabulary in the directional task is thoroughly understood.

1.4.n.1   Directional tasks involve vocabulary comprehension in sentences. Words themselves such as 'on, over, under,' may be misunderstood as well as parts of words, such as 'es, ing, and ed.'

AUDITION

Techniques for Curriculum Adaptation	Extra Information, Materials or References

1.5 **The child does not "use" sound appropriately** (also child tends to ignore sound).

1.5.a Encourage the child to listen to the radio or tape recorded music during free time.

1.5.a.1 Begin by having the child simply listen to music which can tap a different part of the brain from the language related areas. From there, initiate simple sound identification games and activities. A full regimen of sound awareness, sound identification, rhythm, and sound sequence activities can be started. Continue with other sound basics such as memory and discrimination tasks. Numerous activities and books emphasizing these skills are available on the market.

1.5.b Provide the child with numerous activities in which sound is dominant. Comment on the sounds heard.

1.5.b.1 Activities in which sound can be classified into categories is helpful. Make sound charts for their categories, such as animal sounds, vehicle sounds, etc.

1.5.b.2 Make use of sound stories. Have the child see that sounds are always around us and that we constantly make use of them. Stress the importance of them in our everyday lives.

1.5.b.3 The child can make better 'use' of sound when he/she begins to know sound better. The sounds must make sense to his/her world. During times of fluctuating hearing loss, the child's sound world was/is not stabilized so that he/she is not making use appropriately of the input messages.

Techniques for Curriculum Adaptation	Extra Information, Materials or References

1.5   The child does not "use" sound appropriately (also child tends to ignore sound). (Continued)

	1.5.b.4 Let the child physically experience as many sounds as possible. Instead of just isolating certain sounds, such as "that is a cow," include other accompanying sounds such as "I hear the cow mooing. His tail is swishing. His ear wiggled. Several flies are buzzing around him." Provide the child with as much information as possible about the sound. When children are learning how sounds are useful, they take in all the meanings associated with one sound.
1.5.c Provide other sensory input when initiating an auditory activity.	1.5.c.1 By stimulating the other senses, the auditory input can be stressed so that the brain has time to assimilate the information.
1.5.d Provide sound field amplification.	1.5.d.1 By providing louder sound input, the stimulus being received may have input now, whereas before, when hearing was diminished or inconsistent, the sound was not important and therefore, the child may have learned to 'not use' or 'turn off' sound. The amplified sound stimulates the brain so that the child can become aware of the meaning and importance of sound.
	1.5.d.2 See 1.1.d

AUDITION

Techniques for Curriculum Adaptation	Extra Information, Materials or References

1.5 **The child does not "use" sound appropriately** (also child tends to ignore sound). (Continued)

1.5.e Use sound enhancement system especially during activities where sound is important.	1.5.e.1 Although all sound is important and has subtle meanings to every situation, the amplification of sound during specific segments of instruction can emphasize a weak skill area for the child.
	1.5.e.2 See 1.1.o
1.5.f Use personal sound amplification with a child who needs constant sound amplification to become more aware of his/her environment.	1.5.f.1 See 1.1.n
	1.5.f.2 This method might be less costly than sound field amplification because only one unit is used. It can be used continuously with the child who needs to make better use of his/her sound input.
1.5.g Encourage the child to "use the eyes to help the ears."	1.5.g.1 See Curriculum Adaptation section.
	1.5.g.2 The child may be more visually oriented. For the child to learn what sounds are and how they can be important, he/she may need to see the sound being made or have a visual representation such as a picture to stimulate recognition of the sound.
1.5.h For the older child, provide reference points for remembering how certain sounds are useful and important.	1.5.h.1 For example, pictures, objects, activities, written cues, outlines can be helpful. They help direct the focus of the sound through other senses. Then support the idea with verbal input.

Techniques for Curriculum Adaptation	Extra Information, Materials or References

1.5 **The child does not "use" sound appropriately** (also child tends to ignore sound). (Continued)

1.5.h.2 An example: print an outline for fire emergencies. This may sound commonplace but very often the otitis media affected child will simply follow the activities of the other children. The teacher can write down the steps to follow. Use diagrams for the smaller children. Go over the chart with each successive fire drill. The child is given the reference point of going over, seeing the words or pictures and triggering what to do in the fire drill. The child may hear the fire drill and can tell you perhaps what the sound is but may not be able to go beyond that except by followng others.

1.5.i When introducing a new topic, emphasize stress patterns within sentences.

1.5.i.1 Very often subtle stress changes within sentences are missed. For example, if the child heard "Mary only took two crayons," versus "Mary only took two crayons," the child may miss the subtle distinctions. This is very important when teaching new ideas, because the idea that the teacher is trying to get across may come out totally different for the child because of the subtle misinterpretations.

1.5.i.2 Inflections of words can be missed as well. For example, "You did what?" where the last part of 'what' is raised significantly and means that the person can't believe it, versus "You did what?" where the last part of 'what' is hardly raised at all and means please repeat what you said, can have significant impact on what the child is comprehending.

AUDITION

Techniques for Curriculum Adaptation	Extra Information, Materials or References

1.5 **The child does not "use" sound appropriately** (also child tends to ignore sound). (Continued)

1.5.j Provide numerous opportunities to develop classification skills.	1.5.j.1 Classification skills can eventually aid in the development of organizational skills. They help the child put things in their place. They can also lead toward development of skills which will help the child eliminate non-essential cues and organize essential sound cues.

1.6 **The child says "huh" or "what" frequently.**

1.6.a See 2.2	1.6.a.1 This problem area is listed under two objectives because it can fit both objective areas. Cognition is the knowledge base of learning. It is drawn from sensory information and allows the child to make sense of his/her environment. When the child is either not hearing, not understanding, or not processing the incoming message, it affects the cognitive function as well as the auditory function. The auditory function is the ability to receive auditory input and make use of it appropriately.

1.7 **The child has a short attention span.**

1.7.a Provide a variety of activities utilizing many different presentation methods for teaching one unit.	1.7.a.1 Sometimes it is easiest simply to sit and talk with children to teach a topic. The otitis media affected child may have great difficulty with this because his/her attention span may not last for more than a few minutes.

Techniques for Curriculum Adaptation	Extra Information, Materials or References

1.7   The child has a short attention span. (Continued)

	1.7.a.2 Talk for a few minutes, then change the presentation mode. Use hands-on activities, visual displays such as pictures, books and charts, listening activities, child involvement, etc. Provide as many different modes as possible. This requires more preparation on the part of the teacher, but the effects are very worthwhile.
1.7.b Try simplifying the language you are using.	1.7.b.1 Sometimes the child's "short attention span" can be caused by the language which is beyond the child's comprehension abilities. If he/she is not comprehending or processing the information, then his/her behavior response may be one of not attending, either by physical movement, verbal response, or not responding.
	1.7.b.2 Don't assume that the child understands the language being used. He/she may understand 90% of what is being said but the 10% that he/she doesn't understand may be frustrating enough to turn the child off to listening, hence the "short attention span."
1.7.c Small group instruction or individual instruction for key subjects may be the best way to extend the attention span.	1.7.c.1 The extraneous influences such as noise, visual distractors, and verbal interactions can seriously affect the child's ability to attend to what is happening in the classroom. Small group or individual instruction can be structured so that the extraneous influences are minimized.

AUDITION

Techniques for Curriculum Adaptation	Extra Information, Materials or References

1.7   The child has a short attention span. (Continued)

1.7.d Provide amplification which will increase the intensity of sound sensations the child receives.	1.7.d.1 Often with the increase in sound, the child finds it easier to attend because the sound input source is blocking out the other disturbances.The auditory input is being emphasized.
	1.7.d.2 Sound field amplification, personal sound amplification, and sound enhancement systems are all ways to provide the increased amplification. This amplification should be monitored initially by someone such as the educational audiologist who can ensure that appropriate levels of amplification are maintained. However the classroom teacher can then easily learn how to monitor the equipment.
	1.7.d.3 The increased amplification allows more of the auditory message to be heard. The inflections, stress patterns, voice quality, intonations, etc. are heard and, with time, the linguistic message may take on more importance.
	1.7.d.4 Ensure that the sound is not distorted, but simply amplified.
1.7.e Try teaching or discussing less subject matter at one sitting time. Vary the length of the time for presentations.	1.7.e.1 Try interspersing a variety of activities so that the child can work at extending his/her listening behaviors.

Techniques for Curriculum Adaptation	Extra Information, Materials or References

1.7 The child has a short attention span. (Continued)

1.7.f Discuss work objectives with child. Develop a time-on-task chart from which child can monitor his/her attending.

1.7.f.1 Set the boundaries of acceptable versus unacceptable behavior. This can work more appropriately with the older child, but can also be readily adapted for the younger child.

1.7.f.2 The child is ultimately responsible for his/her own actions. The short attention span may be something that can be worked on by behavior charts. However, it's important to remember that while the child is straining to extend the attention span, little learning may occur. This may be because the child is directing all his/her energy into attending. There is little energy left for absorbing the information presented.

1.7.g Try varying the delivery mode of the information.

1.7.g.1 Sometimes by altering the auditory input, the child is given more cues by which to receive the message. It also gives his/her processing center a break. Try lengthening pauses, change the prosody (the rhythmic aspect of language), and group ideas together. This will allow the child extra processing time and help in the organization of the language units.

1.7.h Make sure the listening environment has appropriate acoustics.

1.7.h.1 When extra sound is reverberating or echoing the child may have great difficulty attending to a task.

1.7.h.2 Walls, room size, sound absorbing materials, placement of furniture, and people in the room all must be considered. The acoustic environment can be restructured. For more information on acoustics in the

AUDITION

Techniques for Curriculum Adaptation	Extra Information, Materials or References

1.7 **The child has a short attention span.** (Continued)

	classroom, see Berg (1987); and Ross (1972)
	1.7.h.3 Eliminate extraneous sounds when possible. Turn off motor noise. With groups teach away from the heater or fish tank. This can greatly enhance the child's attention capabilities.

1.8 **The child appears to have a delayed response to sound.**

1.8.a Provide the child with enough time to respond.	1.8.a.1 Frequently, the teacher expects immediate responses. The otitis media affected child may need extra time to process what he/she has heard, figure out a response, and then respond. To encourage the child to respond and not just give up when he/she can't proceed fast enough, let him/her know that he/she will be allowed to finish his/her thought process and come up with an answer.
	1.8.a.2 Sometimes, while waiting for a response, another thought can be introduced to the rest of the group. For example, the teacher might say "John, I'm going to give you some time to think about your answer. I'm very interested in what you're going to say. While you're thinking, I'm going to show a picture of the inside of the ship. (Pause) OK, John, have you figured out if this ship is a clipper or a schooner? (Pause for response.) Great! You thought that out nicely."

Techniques for Curriculum Adaptation	Extra Information, Materials or References

1.8   The child appears to have a delayed response to sound. (Continued)

1.8.b   With linguistic related input, try altering the rate of speech.

1.8.b.1   Processing the verbal message may be easier for the child if the rate of speech is slower (but not enough to be distorted), if pauses are lengthened, and if ideas are grouped in smaller units.

1.8.c   Amplification can provide an extra stimulus for processing sound.

1.8.c.1   Sometimes the child simply needs to have his auditory sense stimulated. If the child's hearing was inconsistent during his/her growing years, he/she may need the extra input to promote new learning of the sounds in the environment.

1.8.c.2   Personal sound amplifiers, sound field amplification and sound enhancement systems can be helpful depending on the particular situation. Sound field amplification is helpful for the whole class, especially when many of the children have otitis media histories. Personal sound amplification amplifies all the noise and will be best in quieter situations. Sound enhancement systems can block out extraneous noise for direct input.

1.8.d   Be aware that the child may not have processed the entire message. The delay may actually be one of confusion over the message received.

1.8.d.1   Sometimes repeating the exact sentence followed by the same message rephrased can help the child feel more positive about the message received and about what answer to formulate. The hesitation or delay may be the child's lack of confidence in his/her ability to respond.

AUDITION

Techniques for Curriculum Adaptation	Extra Information, Materials or References

1.8   The child appears to have a delayed response to sound. (Continued)

1.8.e   When the child does not seem to respond to environmental sounds until a few seconds later, encourage him/her to notice and respond to the sound more appropriately by providing extra cues or verbal input.

1.8.e.1   For example, if the child does not hear a buzzer in the school indicating a special activity, the sound should be commented on while it is happening. Stir the child's mind to be aware of the sound while it is happening.

1.8.f   Be aware that environmental noise (ambient noise) and reverberation can distort sound. It may also lead to over-stimulation of the child's sensory input.

1.8.f.1   Try to ensure proper acoustics in the classroom if possible.

1.9   The child is a slow task starter.

1.9.a   Provide ways to develop the child's self confidence.

1.9.a.1   Very often the child does not trust himself/herself with what he/she has heard. Therefore, have the child look at what others are doing before starting, to corroborate what he/she processed with what should be done. The child is afraid to take the chance of starting something and being wrong. He/she does not want to experience failure.

1.9.a.2   Allow the child to ask for clarification of the task at hand. Otitis media affected children are often afraid to ask for clarification because of the failure they have experienced in the past. The teacher needs to work for positive self interaction with the child.

Techniques for Curriculum Adaptation	Extra Information, Materials or References

1.9   The child is a slow task starter. (Continued)

	1.9.a.3 Often the otitis media affected child portrays a "negative" child. Because his/her"spoiled-child like" behaviors, some people turn away from wanting to react positively with the child. However, the child needs to have his/her self confidence raised in new, linguistically difficult situations, in order for the "negative" behavior to change. Look beyond these behaviors to understanding the whys of the behavior and react from there. The child's negative self concept can be acted out in so many different ways – being afraid to start a task without being sure, pouting, shouting, overactivity, etc.
1.9.b Allow the child to have a buddy who can be asked to clarify verbal instruction.	1.9.b.1 The buddy can allow the child to not feel inadequate by having to ask the teacher for clarification. Some children do not feel comfortable asking the teacher for extra input. Other children feel special if they are allowed to ask for clarification. Asking a friend or classmate can be less threatening.
	1.9.b.2 An NCR copy of notes or homework is a useful tool for the older child. 'Notetakers' and 'Hear-U Notes' are two published forms of these tools.

AUDITION

Techniques for Curriculum Adaptation	Extra Information, Materials or References

1.9   The child is a slow task starter. (Continued)

1.9.c Provide positive reactions or "strokes" when the child begins to start task immediately.	1.9.c.1 Begin with an activity that appears linguistically and auditorily easy for the child. Discuss and encourage starting the task quickly and promptly. Praise the child if he/she does. This pattern may need to be repeated many times before the child internalizes it. Sometimes, the otitis media affected child appears to take a longer time to internalize something before he/she feels good about carrying it through. Occasionally, the patterns are so set that they can never be changed.
1.9.d Provide the child with a way to remember the task at hand.	1.9.d.1 The teacher can provide verbal or visual clues that can help the child start the task. Frequently, directions are given in a group. The child can give the direction verbally while in the group and may be able initially to repeat the direction at his/her desk, but his/her thoughts then go elsewhere. The teacher can develop constructive work skill levels for the whole class. For example: Step 1, listen for the directions, repeat the directions; Step 2: go to your desk, get proper equipment and start the direction; Step 3: when finished, put the papers in the bins. If the child has trouble starting, the teacher can bring his/her attention back to the task by saying, "John, Step 2." To avoid singling out the child, the teacher could say, "Everyone should be at Step 2." If the child still doesn't start, a "2" can be placed on his/her desk.

Techniques for Curriculum Adaptation	Extra Information, Materials or References

1.9   **The child is a slow task starter.** (Continued)

1.9.e   Structure organizational skills for the whole class but, in particular, for the otitis media affected child.

1.9.e.1   Often the otitis media affected child needs total structure to function adequately. If an instruction is given in one place, and then the child goes to another place, his/her internal structure is disrupted. The step method in 1.9.d.1 is one way to accomplish the necessary structure.

Another way is to walk the child through a pictorial method of what steps to do with class instructions. This may seem to be a waste of time, but often the child needs to have the extra clues for organization so that his/her world makes more sense. If the child feels comfortable with his/her world, he/she will function better.

1.9.f   After allowing assimilation time, provide the child with options for task completion.

1.9.f.1   If the child feels that by completing the task, he/she will receive something beneficial, he/she may start the task. For example: if playtime is allowed after the task, the child might initiate the task faster than if he/she knew another paper and pencil task were to follow. With options, the child can choose to finish and play versus not finish and miss playtime.

1.9.f.2   Sometimes having the child track his/her options can be helpful. The child may not be aware of how many times he/she chooses not to play. The child may blame the teacher for not being able to play, but in this way, can become aware of the results of his/her own options. The responsibility is placed squarely upon the child.

AUDITION

Techniques for Curriculum Adaptation	Extra Information, Materials or References

1.9   The child is a slow task starter. (Continued)

1.9.g   The task may simply seem overwhelming to the child. Provide steps to completions which break down the whole task into parts. As the child accomplishes one part, he/she takes a giant step toward total completion.

1.9.g.1   Very often, the child can do small tasks but large tasks are too much. The thought of starting a larger task can be frightening. What makes a 'large' task to this child may be miniscule to the teacher. For example, doing one line on a worksheet with four items may be too many items for the child's internal comfort. He/she needs to feel comfortable initiating the task. To avoid the task, the child will talk, move, think, stare, sit, or do anything to avoid taking the first step.

1.9.g.2   Provide steps to success. For example: tell the child to do one row and then bring it to the teacher. This extra little input may give him/her the impetus and courage to proceed. Another way would be to block out the bottom of the page with a card while doing the top row and then proceed down the page. The structure for completion has been provided.

1.9.h   Classroom amplification or some other form of amplification may be necessary to ensure that proper input of the auditory message was received.

1.9.h.1   Sometimes, the child is simply unsure of what the directional task was. Because of this unsurety, the child will delay starting the task until he/she is sure or is ready to gamble and guess. The amplification provides a slight boost to the auditory message which sometimes makes the message more comprehensible.

Techniques for Curriculum Adaptation	Extra Information, Materials or References

1.9   The child is a slow task starter. (Continued)

1.9.i   Ensure that the language in the directional task is not too difficult.

1.9.i.1   The child may simply need time to figure out the language of what was directed. Simple, direct language is best. What might seem simple to a teacher, may be confusing to the child. For example: the child may have great confusion over irregular verb tenses due to the lack of hearing when his/her language was emerging. Plurals also can create problems. When using these forms, stop and consider whether the child is simply confused over the language of the directional task.

1.9.i.2   Although some plurals and irregular verb tense difficulty may seem age appropriate, the child with otitis media should be evaluated more closely to see how the effect of the confusions affect his/her everyday functioning. See Hasenstab, 1987, *Language Learning and Otitis Media.*

1.10   The child fails to complete assigned tasks.

1.10.a   Provide steps to completion. Structure activities into small segments which will allow a progression to the end. Build up to longer tasks gradually.

1.10.a.1   See 1.9.g

1.10.b   Allow the child to have a classroom buddy to whom he/she can go for clarification.

1.10.b.1   See 1.9.b

AUDITION

Techniques for Curriculum Adaptation	Extra Information, Materials or References
1.10 **The child fails to complete assigned tasks.** (Continued)	
1.10.c Provide the child with a "break" time in the middle of an assignment if it gets too much for him/her.	1.10.c.1 By breaking the time spent at the task into two parts, the child can sometimes accomplish more. For example, for some children, allowing them to stand and stretch when they're halfway through a task, allows them to involve other modalities. The simple activity from the physical input of moving may allow them to complete the directional task since it often seems to be less threatening or seemingly impossible.
1.10.d Provide ways to bolster the child's self concept.	1.10.d.1 See 1.9.a
	1.10.d.2 The child may feel that he/she functions best as a failure so that by not completing his/her assignments the child is fulfilling the picture of himself/herself. By developing positive responses to finishing work, he/she may be able to get beyond this feeling of failure. This cannot happen overnight. Frequently, even though the child has been provided with numerous times to succeed, if he/she does not finish one day for whatever reason, the one negative reaction is more potent than many positives. It is important to constantly encourage the positive. Allow the child to feel good about himself/herself.
1.10.e Expand the child's auditory memory skills abilities.	1.10.e.1 See 1.9.d

Techniques for Curriculum Adaptation	Extra Information, Materials or References

1.10   The child fails to complete assigned tasks. (Continued)

	1.10.e.2 Sometimes, the child can remember the first part of an assignment and can begin it right away or delay it slightly. However, when halfway through, he/she may simply forget what comes next. If the child does not feel good enough about asking for further clarification from a teacher or a "buddy", then he/she frequently just stops doing the task and leaves it uncompleted.
	1.10.e.3 One way to help the child to remember the task at hand is to have him/her report the direction as soon as you give it, then repeat it silently while doing the task.
	1.10.c.4 Using the technique of "eyes to help your ears" while giving the direction can also help the child make use of other sensory information from which to draw. The visual input can trigger the memory for what was to have been accomplished.
1.10.f Establish a contract with the child to finish his/her work.	1.10.f.1 Develop a clear understanding of intent toward accomplishing a goal. Have both teacher and student work towards the accomplishment. If the child verbalizes that he/she just doesn't want to do it, then you need to help the child establish the groundwork for good work habits.

AUDITION

Techniques for Curriculum Adaptation	Extra Information, Materials or References

1.11   The child has difficulty hearing differences between sounds or phonemes.

1.11.a   Sound field amplification can provide extra sensory input to make the sounds more distinguishable.

1.11.a.1   Often the children have normal hearing except when they are functioning with a current episode of otitis media. The children are having difficulty hearing the sound differences because of the time during their development when their hearing was fluctuating. They are unsure of what they are hearing. The amplification provides a slight extra intensity to stimulate the auditory centers. It is important that the sound is not distorted as can happen with raised voices.

1.11.b   Provide a reference point if talking about pictures, objects, activities, etc.

1.11.b.1   The children may not hear the differences between two similar sounding words. It is helpful to provide an object to help the children with an extra input mode. In effect they are "using the eyes to help their ears" decipher what they heard. It helps them direct their focus through their other senses and helps support the verbal input.

1.11.c   Provide an acoustically appropriate environment.

1.11.c.1   Background and environmental noise can mask out finite sound differences. The child tends to make more errors in discrimination when the sounds he/she needed to hear were overlapped by extraneous sounds.

1.11.c.2   Classroom seating can improve listening skills. Seat the child away from doors, windows, fans and busy activity areas when doing group work.

Techniques for Curriculum Adaptation	Extra Information, Materials or References

1.11 **The child has difficulty hearing differences between sounds or phonemes.** (Continued)

	1.11.c.3 Phonemes may be perceived in quiet or isolation. However, they may not be perceived adequately when in noise or when they are presented rapidly.
	1.11.c.4 Transitional information may be lost and fricatives in the final position may also be missed when noise levels in the classroom are not adequate. (Reichman & Healey, 1983)
	1.11.c.5 The child may miss out on high frequency fricatives. Brief utterances and high frequency information may be lost (Doble & Berlin, 1979)
1.11.d Emphasize visual coding and decoding directly to the meaning of words.	1.11.d.1 Sounds in isolation may have little or no meaning for the otitis media affected child. Teaching the whole word with visual emphasis may prove helpful.
1.11.e If the child misarticulates a word, say the correct word again in a related sentence with a slight voice intensity emphasis.	1.11.e.1 The child frequently feels uncomfortable and sometimes inadequate with his/her communication skills. By repeating the correct word again with a slightly raised, voiced emphasis on that word, the child is attending and hears the sound again. He/she may try to self-correct the word either internally or verbally.
	1.11.e.2 Don't correct the errors the child makes. Provide enough references to train his/her ears to the correctly produced sound. The correction should come from within.

AUDITION

Techniques for Curriculum Adaptation	Extra Information, Materials or References

1.11   The child has difficulty hearing differences between sounds or phonemes. (Continued)

	1.11.e.3 The Speech Language Pathologist should evaluate the child's misarticulations if this is questioned.
1.11.f Consider the type of phoneme and sound errors being made and provide extra help when they are low intensity sounds.	1.11.f.1 The child with otitis media frequently has difficulty distinguishing low intensity words like a, an, the, on and up. They often focus in on nouns, verbs, adjectives and adverbs.
	1.11.f.2 Unstressed phonemes and words are often missed.
1.11.g Teach in a stationary position.	1.11.g.1 Moving around the room alters how the child perceives sound. The teacher's head may be turned away from him/her so the child may only receive a portion of the sound input message. The sound is going away from him versus towards his/her ears. If the teacher then turns around the child receives some of the message, but not all the message clearly, thereby creating confusion.
	1.11.g.2 Sound field amplification and sound enhancement systems eliminate the need for this. The teacher has the freedom of mobility.
1.11.h When teaching reading, use a multi sensory method.	1.11.h.1 A method that gives visual, auditory and tactile clues for comprehension can be helpful. *The Open Court System* is one such method.
1.11.i The child may always have difficulty with this task so try alternative techniques.	1.11.i.1 It can be helpful to teach meaningful phrase units instead of single sounds or words.

Techniques for Curriculum Adaptation	**Extra Information, Materials or References**

1.12   The child has difficulty understanding and repeating words of many syllables or sounds. Common error words are: spaghetti/pasghetti and animal/aminal/amimal.

1.12.a Provide activities for listening to three or more sounds.	1.12.a.1 Frequently, the child has difficulty hearing the differences among many sounds. Start with simple environmental sounds and then build gradually to the more complex sounds of phonemes and syllables. It is helpful to start with two sounds and have the idea and experience well-embedded before introducing three sounds. This may also provide a quick reference point to see where the child's breakdown point is.
	1.12.a.2 For example, to start, take what is called a "sound story." These can be concocted in class or can be purchased. A two sound story could be the teacher walking into the classroom (where sound is heard, not on carpeting) and turning on the light switch. The child works through the meaning and auditory experience of the whole situation. This can be expanded to the teacher saying "Good morning class."
	1.12.a.3 The exercises can be extended to include phonemes or syllables. Start with a separation of the sounds and then blend them. Often the child has difficulty with the individual phonemes. Begin with two sounds and them progress to three or more. Frequently, the breakdown occurs with three items or sounds.

AUDITION

Techniques for Curriculum Adaptation	Extra Information, Materials or References
1.12	The child has difficulty understanding and repeating words of many syllables or sounds. Common error words are: spaghetti/pasghetti and animal/aminal/amimal. (Continued)	

1.12.b	Encourage activities that deal with rhythm.	1.12.b.1	Rhythm can influence the flow of a word. The rhythm of a word can alter how the child perceives inflections, pitch, intensity, and durations of the sounds. Faster rhythms of words such as 'animal' may make it more difficult for the child to hear, perceive, and reproduce the word.
		1.12.b.2	With activities that provide physical, visual, and auditory modalities, the reception centers are being stimulated simultaneously. Input is being received and may be retained better.
		1.12.b.3	Saying syllables and phonemes to a musical rhythm can be helpful to some children. Again, different parts of the brain are working together to accomplish the desired result.
1.12.c	Provide activities for developing auditory sequential memory tasks.	1.12.c.1	The child might have difficulty putting three items together. Begin the practice with gross objects or sounds, then gradually work toward individual sounds and eventually to syllables. It might be easier, before working on individual sounds, to work on sequencing words. The word may have more meaning for the child.

Techniques for Curriculum Adaptation	Extra Information, Materials or References

1.12   The child has difficulty understanding and repeating words of many syllables or sounds. Common error words are: spaghetti/pasghetti and animal/aminal/amimal. (Continued)

1.12.d   Try to provide consistent intonation patterns, inflection and stress patterns during connected speech.

1.12.d.1   The child functions best with consistency. When getting him/her to hear words, a consistent speech pattern allows him/her to listen, perceive and comprehend the message a little bit easier.

1.12.e   Provide opportunities to practice contrasts and similarities, especially with individual sounds and words.

1.12.e.1   Rhyming is a skill that can be useful.

1.12.e.2   "Odd-man-out" is a game where words are presented. Two are the same and one is different. Have the child identify those that are alike or those that are different.

1.12.e.3   Having the child listen for the differences and similarities can allow the child to internalize what he hears when he says a word incorrectly, such as "pasghetti" and eventually to self-correct it.

Techniques for Curriculum Adaptation	Extra Information, Materials or References

2.1.   The child learns better through senses other than auditory.

2.1.a   Build upon other senses that are strong while also emphasizing the auditory sense. The technique of using the "eyes to help the ears" is useful here.

2.1.a.1   The technique of using "eyes to help the ears" is explained earlier in the book in the objective information.

2.1.b   Provide as many varied input and output modes as possible. Use body gestures. Visual aids can also provide extra input.

2.1.b.1   As the child "listens" better, control the amount of input by the other senses to strengthen the child's auditory sense.

2.1.b.2   As an example: If the teacher is having a lesson about ships and shipbuilding, include props like boats, masts, sails, ropes, etc., and use pictures to visually represent the item. Likewise, use the sounds of boats in water – include the sounds of the workmen or sailors, too. The child can hear and feel the items and come up with a total experience.

2.1.c   When possible, break down the components of your teaching lesson. Provide as many hands on or visual portions as you can. Encourage the children to watch you during the auditory portions.

2.1.d   Use sound field amplification. This stresses hearing the teacher's voice over extraneous noise, thereby triggering children's auditory sense into greater use.

2.1.d.1   See the research on Project M.A.R.R.S. for information on the effectiveness of sound field amplification. (See Ray, et al, 1984)

COGNITION

Techniques for Curriculum Adaptation	Extra Information, Materials or References

2.1. The child learns better through senses other than auditory. (Continued)

2.1.e Adapt spelling lessons to whole word units instead of individual sounds within words. The child will respond better to the sight word versus having to learn to spell through mastery of the sounds of the words. If possible, teach words that have meaning to the child first, to build his/her confidence.

2.1.e.1 Spelling is often an area that is difficult for this child because the sounds within the word are confusing. Having to put sounds together to form a word is stressful for him or her.

2.1.f Enhance the auditory with other senses. When a direction is given, have the child repeat it verbally. This is easy in a one-on-one situation. In a large group, teach the child to quietly repeat the instruction to himself/herself. The physical task of repeating it aloud (pulling it from immediate memory) and re-hearing or re-thinking it stimulates the additional recall of the information. Avoid calling on the child in a group to verbally repeat a direction. The child often doesn't feel comfortable with his/her input system, and can't repeat the direction without feeling belittled. Very often, this will turn the child off so that he or she will not want to respond verbally in the future.

2.1.f.1 The actual physical follow through of verbally repeating the direction triggers a kinesthetic response in combination with the auditory response.

2.1.f.2 See Luria (1970)

2.1.f.3 Enhance the child's self image as often as you can. Don't call on the child in circumstances where he or she feels uncomfortable. That way, he or she can place more emphasis on listening and understanding instead of having the fear or stress of being called upon block the learning process.

2.1.g Use visual reinforcers whenever possible. For young children, visual representation through pictures can stimulate recall. The older child can benefit from words or sentences written as reminders.

Techniques for Curriculum Adaptation	Extra Information, Materials or References

2.1. **The child learns better through senses other than auditory.** (Continued)

2.1.h   Reduce class and teacher motor activities when stressing auditory input, such as during discussions.

2.1.h.1   A child can attend to a stationary person better than to one who is moving because of the reduction in the stimulation of the visual center. A child also will retain more when no extraneous activity is in progress during auditory input, such as in discussions.

2.1.i   Record lessons and instructions on tape so that the child can hear the material repeated at a later time.

2.1.i.1   The extra benefit of listening again to what is presented during aural instructions can allow the child to: 1) rehearse the input in his/her mind; 2) re-experience the thought; and 3) re-think or piece together what he/she thinks was said. The child can do so without feeling afraid to take a chance and fail — thus, can feel success, which helps build up a positive self-concept.

2.2 **The child says "huh" or "what" frequently.**

2.2.a   Repeat the message to provide additional input for the child. Make sure the entire phrase is repeated exactly how it was said and not what you thought was the important part.

2.2.a.1   The child often hears the important part of the message but misses out on the sub parts. For the child to feel comfortable in a response, all the pieces of the message need to make sense. Therefore, exact repetition is important the first time. Rephrasing can be done immediately after the exact repetition in case the original vocabulary or sentence structure was too difficult for the child to comprehend.

2.2.b   If the child says 'what?' a second time, then rephrase the original message to provide additional input.

COGNITION

Techniques for Curriculum Adaptation	Extra Information, Materials or References

2.2 **The child says "huh" or "what" frequently.** (Continued)

2.2.c   Make sure you have the child's attention before speaking to allow for maximum message input.

2.2.d   Allow the child more processing time: use a slower rate of speech, but don't distort; lengthen your pauses; group meaningful word units; but continue to use regular voice quality and rhythm.

2.2.e Minimize extraneous background noise whenever possible.	2.2.e.1 Background noise can mask out sounds within words. The child may perceive a word other than the one spoken and it does not make sense to him or her in the context heard. He or she then says 'huh?' to clarify the meaning of the misperceived word.
2.2.f Sound field amplification allows the teacher's voice to be heard over extraneous noise and provides a more direct input. The child has less difficulty hearing the sounds within sentences.	2.2.f.1 The teacher does not have to be so concerned with the direction of his/her voice. His/her voice comes out through the speaker amplified for everyone.
2.2.g If sound field amplification is not available, obtaining eye contact with the child is helpful in order to assist listening with visual input, such as seeing the sounds of the words spoken on the speaker's face. The child is having his "eyes help his ears."	

Techniques for Curriculum Adaptation	Extra Information, Materials or References

2.2   The child says "huh"or "what"frequently. (Continued)

2.2.h   In a one-on-one situation, having the child repeat what he/she thinks was said is helpful. It is a good way to find out the child's miscues.

2.2.h.1   Frequently, a child says "huh?" but has understood most of it and pieced together the thought from previously stored information. The child may not trust himself/herself in trying the response until sure of the input message. In a one-to-one situation when the child has been asked to repeat the statement, praise the child for having successfully heard and repeated the message. Next, encourage the child to follow through appropriately. Additionally, praise the child for following through on his/her own. Praise should be meaningful and not overdone.

2.2.i   Keep questions simple; avoid lengthy, multiple part questions.

2.2.i.1   Very often, the children have difficulty with auditory sequence memory. In addition to not comprehending long tasks, they may forget more than the first or second part of questions, or they may remember only the first or the last item.

2.2.j   Use visual aids whenever possible. Incorporate the other body senses to enhance the verbal message.

2.2.j.1   Having been deprived of auditory input at various times in their development, their other senses may be more enhanced but are not always trained. Encourage eye usage whenever feasible. As the children grow older, the specialist may want to decrease their dependency on other senses and try to further develop their auditory sense.

COGNITION

Techniques for Curriculum Adaptation	Extra Information, Materials or References

2.2   The child says "huh" or "what" frequently. (Continued)

2.2.k   Make sure your voice is directed towards the child's face. Do not look around or turn your head as this will distort the sound going to his/her ear. Very often, the child has difficulty piecing together the rhythm of speech, the inflection of the voice and the pitch of the voice into a meaningful message.

2.3   The child needs extra processing time.

2.3.a   In presenting ideas or information to the child, alter the rate of speech: lengthen the pauses between the sentences, group ideas together, change the prosody or accent of the voice. This allows the child's brain to organize the incoming message more appropriately.

2.3.a.1   Due to intermittent auditory input during the formative first two years of life, the child may need additional processing time for the necessary organizational input of the language units and the particular speech sounds.

2.3.a.2   Due to the lack of sufficient stimuli in early years, the child may have subtle difficulties with the duration, frequency, timbre and prosody of sounds. This would account for the difficulty the child has in comprehending certain sentences.

2.3.b   The sentence or passage that the child listened to may have been linguistically too complicated for him/her to process. Qualify what was said. Perhaps you can delete certain aspects of the sentence.

Techniques for Curriculum Adaptation	Extra Information, Materials or References

2.3   **The child needs extra processing time.** (Continued)

2.3.c   While allowing the child time to process the idea, restate exactly the same idea. This gives the child even more input so that if all of the idea was not perceived the first time, the second message repeats the information.

2.3.d   After restating the idea, rephrase or expand upon the idea.

2.3.d.1   This allows you to modify any linguistic difficulties in the original statement.

2.3.e   Allow for more total sensory experience with the concept, idea or sentence constructs that were difficult for the child to process.

2.3.e.1   Frequently the child simply needs more experience with the concept being expressed, either verbally or manipulatively. The child may simply need more experience with processing a certain language structure such as plural word forms for the child to make sense of the input. For example, if the teacher asked the child to mark the picture with the ducks and his/her choices were a picture of one duck or of three ducks, he/she may simply be having difficulty figuring out what was heard.

2.3.f   Encourage the child to ask questions to clarify what he/she heard.

2.3.f.1   Very often the child is simply confused between what he/she thought was heard and what he/she apparently thinks the teacher said. The child may have heard a sentence such as "Mark the cat with the dot," as "Park the gas with the top" and be very confused. These listening errors may be caused by the place, manner and voicing characteristics of the speech sounds within the sentence.

COGNITION

Techniques for Curriculum Adaptation	Extra Information, Materials or References

2.3 **The child needs extra processing time.** (Continued)

2.3.g	Use of sound field amplification amplifies the signal to noise ratio of the teacher's voice to classroom noise significantly.	2.3.g.1	The extra intensity of the teacher's voice may provide enough additional auditory information so that "processing" may not seem to take as long.
2.3.h	Personal sound amplification can be used in small group or one-on-one situations.	2.3.h.1	See 2.3.g.1
2.3.i	Sound enhancement systems may reduce extraneous noise sufficiently so that the increased auditory signal is better received.	2.3.i.1	See 2.3.g.1
2.3.j	Encourage the child to use a "buddy system."	2.3.j.1	If the child doesn't feel comfortable asking the teacher to clarify what he/she heard, a buddy might be designated to whom the child could go to ask for help and clarification.

2.4 **The child functions best in his/her own orderly world.**

2.4.a	Reduce distraction of extraneous sources when introducing new topic.	2.4.a.1	When the child was initially learning about the auditory world, sound was intermittent and confusing. He/she made sense of the world by creating his/her own sense of order. As sound was not being stimulated at this critical time of development, the child learned to function best by interacting in his/her own world.
		2.4.a.2	More information about sound deprivation can be found in Webster & Webster (1977), Katz (1978).

Techniques for Curriculum Adaptation	Extra Information, Materials or References

2.4   **The child functions best in his/her own orderly world.** (Continued)

2.4.b   Introduce new ideas or activities gradually for this child.

2.4.c   Allow the child to grasp ideas at a slower pace.

    2.4.c.1   After initial introduction of a topic, place articles, objects or pictures in areas where the child can learn through hands on interaction. When you discuss the subject again, the child may respond more appropriately after he/she has had time to "experience" the subject by himself/herself.

2.4.d   Encourage another child to work or play with this child as a way to extend his/her world to others.

2.4.e   When the child is doing seat work, make sure the child has comprehended the directional task so that when working alone, he/she can attempt to follow through.

    2.4.e.1   Sometimes the child can function in his/her own world but that doesn't necessarily correlate with finishing independent work assignments. Frequently the child needs constant encouragement or reinforcement in following through on tasks.

2.4.f   When introducing new ideas, make allowances for inappropriate behavioral responses.

    2.4.f.1   When the child's orderly system is being broken, the child doesn't seem able to accept the new mode easily, thereby creating great internal frustration, anger and conflict. Very often the child responds with crying, tantrums, shouting, or by simply withdrawing.

    2.4.f.2   What may seem inconsequential to the teacher may be monumental to the child's sense of orderliness. For example: the teacher's change from crayons to markers for the class may be extremely disruptive to the child's system. Or on a larger scale, if a

COGNITION

Techniques for Curriculum Adaptation	Extra Information, Materials or References

2.4 The child functions best in his/her own orderly world. (Continued)

	child's seat is changed he/she may react by sulking or behaving negatively. This may be the child's response to a disorderly world rather than the child not liking who he/she is near or where he/she is being seated.
2.4.g Tell the child privately beforehand that some major change will be occurring. If possible, discuss with him why the change should occur. Allow the child to prepare his/her mind-set for the change.	**2.4.g.1** An older child will appreciate the consideration of being prepared for change rather than being surprised by change.

2.5 The child looks at you with a blank confused face.

2.5.a Restate exactly what you said, afterward rephrasing the sentence for extra input.	**2.5.a.1** See 2.3.a.1, 2.3.a.2, 2.3.e.1, 2.3.f.1
2.5.b. The child may benefit from additional experiences with familiar actions, objects, events, or information sources about the topic introduced or about a skill required in the topic. A child can look confused when his/her world is not making sense.	**2.5.b.1** This technique approximates what Piaget says is necessary for Accommodation to occur.
2.5.c Restructure the entire process of the activity in a different manner.	**2.5.c.1** This is easier to do when the child is young. As the child ages, it is harder to break down set ideas and ways.

Techniques for Curriculum Adaptation	Extra Information, Materials or References

2.5 **The child looks at you with a blank confused face.** (Continued)

2.5.d	Analyze the entire activity for the child. Break it down into parts. Discuss the activity in different terms and then put it back together in the original form.	2.5.d.1	Not only does this assist comprehension but enhances vocabulary and other language components such as categorization.
2.5.e	Use sound field amplification.	2.5.e.1	When the signal to noise ratio of the teacher's voice over the background noise is raised significantly, the child may be better able to perceive and interpret the incoming messages.
2.5.f	Personal sound amplification may be used during small group or individual instruction.	2.5.f.1	See 2.5.e.1
2.5.g	Sound enhancement systems may be used effectively in small group instruction.	2.5.g.1	See 2.5.e.1
2.5.h	Expose the child to more of the basic linguistic informational items such as classification, categorization, increased exposure to vocabulary items and object function. With increase in linguistic function, the child may be better able to process the incoming message.	2.5.h.1	The child may not have had enough exposure to the simple language functions which by school age we take for granted. If the child received intermittent confused auditory input in infancy, he/she may not have had enough experience to assimilate the information.
		2.5.h.2	The child may need more help relating objects to particular ideas. He/she may need exposure to meaningful classification. The child has to use his/her senses and clues to arrive at a conclusion. The child's body must learn sense interaction in conjunction with verbal interaction.

COGNITION

Techniques for Curriculum Adaptation	Extra Information, Materials or References

2.5   The child looks at you with a blank confused face. (Continued)

		2.5.h.3	The child may need more exposure to determine the function of objects and may need to discover things that move, things that are light, etc. He/she needs hands-on interaction.
		2.5.h.4	Allow the child time to make generalizations, draw conclusions, and reason logically. Encourage all attempts at this.
2.5.i	Encourage the child to clarify what he/she does not understand.	2.5.i.1	This is easier for the older child but allows the teacher insight into what specific difficulty the child was experiencing.
2.5.j	Decrease the amount of information being given to the child at one time.	2.5.j.1	Sometimes too much information presented all at once may be more than the child can process. If the information is broken down into simpler language structures with simpler vocabulary, at separate intervals, the child may be able to understand what is required.
2.5.k	Decrease the complexity of the message.	2.5.k.1	If the language is broken down to simpler language structures, the child may be able to process the information more easily.
2.5.l	Use a slower rate of speech, lengthen pauses, and group meaningful units within sentences or ideas.	2.5.l.1	By altering the auditory input, processing may be easier.

Techniques for Curriculum Adaptation	Extra Information, Materials or References

2.5 **The child looks at you with a blank confused face. (Continued)**

2.5.m   Use regular voice quality and rhythm while talking.

25m.1   Some children may find some teachers easier to understand than others due to the characteristics of the teacher's voice and rhythm of speech.

25m.2   Men have a lower voice fundamental frequency which may allow these children to "hear" or understand men better than women.

2.6 **The child has difficulty with name recall.**

2.6.1   See 4.1 in its entirety.

2.7 **The child talks around an item or circumlocutes the item instead of giving the vocabulary word**

2.7.1   See 4.1 in its entirety.

2.8 **The child has difficulty with simple questions.**

2.8.a   Expose the child to more basic linguistic information such as classification, categorization, vocabulary.

2.8.a.1   As with all language activities mentioned throughout this guide, enlist the support of the Speech/Language Pathologist.

COGNITION

Techniques for Curriculum Adaptation	Extra Information, Materials or References

2.8   **The child has difficulty with simple questions.** (Continued)

2.8.b	Elongate or over emphasize the rising inflection at the end of a question.	2.8.b.1	Very often when the otitis media affected child was learning to use auditory input, he/she was not hearing adequately to make use of the tonality and inflection of peoples' voices. Therefore, he/she can not interpret or use the rising inflection appropriately to understand a question form.
		2.8.b.2	The child must use past experience for identification of the speech input signal. (Tarnapol, 1971)
		2.8.b.3	The direction of the frequency change of the speech signals what is important for speech sound recognition. (Tarnapol, 1971)
2.8.c	Avoid direct questioning whenever possible, especially with group situations or in noisy environments.	2.8.c.1	For the child who is struggling with his/her communication system, asking a question, giving specific directions or requiring imitations may actually inhibit language use. The child may not feel comfortable enough with his/her language system to venture an answer.
			Very often simple words such as "great!," "uh huh!," "yeah," and "you know" can do more to stimulate language. It is through verbal interaction that language is learned best.
2.8.d	To find out if the child knows the answer to the question, comment on the activity, expand the child's utterances, and discuss the activity with him/her.		

Techniques for Curriculum Adaptation	Extra Information, Materials or References

2.8 The child has difficulty with simple questions. (Continued)

2.8.e Encourage the child to ask for clarification or restatement of the question.

2.8.f Isolating and emphasizing key words in the questions may be helpful. Then expand on the question's topic or rephrase it. An open ended sentence may work better than the question form.

2.8.f.1 For example: If the child is asked, "Where is the ball?" and the child does not respond. The teacher can say, "Ball. The ball is _____. Where is the ball?"

2.8.g Slow the rate of the question down.

2.8.g.1 The child may have difficulty discriminating rapidly presented phonemes. The slower rate may increase comprehension.

2.8.g.2 When the duration of the auditory stimulus increases, the child may process the auditory information more easily.

2.9 The child has difficulty with spelling.

2.9.a Let the child listen to the word to be spelled. Have the child rehearse the phoneme sounds of the work verbally first. Separate the phonemes within the word. Then visually present the word. Have the child blend phonemes together to fit the word initially listened to. Have the child copy the printed form.

2.9.a.1 Luria (1970) noted that when the articulators moved when producing speech, the kinesthetic feedback in conjunction with the auditory feedback enhanced comprehension of the speech sounds.

2.9.a.2 Tarnapol (1971) also indicates the importance of involving the brain's motor analyzer for articulation in speech understanding.

COGNITION

Techniques for Curriculum Adaptation	Extra Information, Materials or References

2.9   The child has difficulty with spelling. (Continued)

2.9.b Choose the spelling feature being taught, e.g. digraphs, diphthong blends or consonants. Have children choose words that they know have those sounds. Each child gives a word verbally to the teacher, who repeats it and writes it on the board. After a list is compiled with as many combinations as possible, the teacher can then choose which will be on the week's spelling list.	2.9.b.1 The visual whole word approach is used. But when the word is chosen at the clue level, the child is allowed input into the formulation of the list with the teacher having the final choice. The child feels as though he/she is involved in a process that used to be difficult. Thinking, hearing and seeing the words involves a different way for the child to initially attack a word.
	2.9.b.2 For example: if working on the oi/oy spelling, children think of words with that sound in it. The teacher then utilizes the words she already may have chosen which were included on the child's list and they are used as the current week's list.
	2.9.b.3 Children are using their own senses to produce the word in their head, saying it auditorily, and then seeing it spelled. A picture can often supplement the activity.
2.9.c If working with a phonetic approach only, incorporate as many other senses for each sound which must be learned.	2.9.c.1 See 4.2.a.1
2.9.d Adapt spelling lessons to whole word units instead of individual sounds within words. The child may respond better to the sight word versus learning through the sounds of the word. If possible, teach words that have meaning to the child so that he/she begins to experience success.	2.9.d.1 Spelling is often one area that causes problems because the sound/letter combinations are difficult for the child to remember. Having to put sounds together to form a word is confusing.

Techniques for Curriculum Adaptation	Extra Information, Materials or References

2.9   The child has difficulty with spelling. (Continued)

2.9.e   When sounding out a word, decrease the amount of time between the separation of sounds, until the sounds almost connect.

2.9.e.1   The child will understand the word better when the word is whole because that's how it has meaning to him.

2.9.e.2   The child usually has difficulty hearing the individual sounds of words when they are in parts. Paradoxically by not separating the sounds, the child may be able to hear the individual sounds.

2.9.f   Instead of a regular written spelling test, a phoneme spelling test may be helpful. Have the child give the word orally in phonemes.

2.9.f.1   This should be done in a quiet environment. The child can often perceive the phoneme in quiet but not if noise is present or the phoneme is rapidly presented.

2.9.g   For practice, put spelling words on a tape. Have the child practice writing the word and then self check with the corresponding words on a ditto sheet.

2.9.h   Make sure the child is able to see the teacher's face during all of the spelling lesson or test.

2.9.h.1   The child may not do well with audition alone but may be better able to figure out the spelling if he/she sees the sound produced and hears the word at the same time.

COGNITION

Techniques for Curriculum Adaptation	Extra Information, Materials or References

2.9   **The child has difficulty with spelling.** (Continued)

2.9.i   Teach the child to see a physical picture of the word in his/her mind. When the child hears the word, he/she is using "the eyes to help the ears".

2.9.j   Analyzing the spelling word may be helpful. Separate the word into parts. Let the child visually see the parts, say them auditorily, feel them with their articulators, discuss them as the separate parts and then integrate them into the whole word. See the whole word, say the word and feel the word.

2.10   **The child has difficulty with mental arithmetic.**

2.10.a Break down the process of the arithmetic problem into parts and explain.	2.10.a.1 The child can be taught letters, numbers and words from visual/auditory presentations, but this does not necessarily mean that he/she comprehends the meaning. This correlates to mental arithmetic because the child needs more hands on activities to comprehend the task.
2.10.b Give the child more opportunity with sorting, classifying, and categorizing objects.	2.10.b.1 Much of mental arithmetic deals with the language concepts which are already weak. The child needs more experiential time to rehearse.
2.10.c Provide sequential memory enrichment activities.	2.10.c.1 Frequently, mental arithmetic problems involve the ability to remember a series of numbers. If a child has sequential memory difficulties, this proves to be troublesome.

Techniques for Curriculum Adaptation	Extra Information, Materials or References

2.11   **The child has difficulty with reading.**

2.11.a   Provide more experiences in exploration, manipulation, and discussion of linguistic material.

2.11.b   Provide more practice with familiar actions, objects, events or information sources.

2.11.c   A modification or change in form may have to take place. Qualify, delete or vary aspects of the language structure. In that way, the child can make better use of the reconstruction of past information to make sense now.

2.11.d   Analyze the process for the child. Separate the problem area into parts, discuss it in different terms and then put it back together.

2.11.e   Increase the exposure to classes and categories. Increased naming practice can be helpful.

2.11.f   Teach letters and words from a visual/auditory presentation. See the letter or word and say the word. Trigger the two senses together.

2.11.b.1   This resembles closely Piaget's Assimilation concept.

2.11.c.1   This resembles closely Piaget's Accommodation.

2.11.c.2   When the child has insufficient information in memory storage to match the language code of the speaker or the written form, he/she is therefore not able to make sense of the content. The only thing the child accomplishes is meaningless reading.

2.11.f.1   Although the letter or word can be memorized, this does not connote understanding.

COGNITION

Techniques for Curriculum Adaptation	Extra Information, Materials or References
2.11 **The child has difficulty with reading.** (Continued)	
2.11.g Isolate key words to be learned. Write them in a special place, such as the blackboard or on a card on the child's desk, as a reference source . Have the child practice the key words by seeing, saying and hearing them altogether.	
1.11.h Teach words through development. Take a reading idea to be taught such as "_at." Have the child formulate all the words that he/she can by adding an initial consonant. The child can make a list of words around that concept which may be easier to remember because he/she formulated it himself/herself.	2.11.h.1 Make sure the child does the work. If done in a large group, the children who respond usually understand the concept already. This list should be developed by teacher and child or buddy and child.
2.11.i Teach whole word units rather than emphasizing hearing the individual sounds within the words. Teaching a whole sentence incorporating the spelling word, if possible, would be even better.	2.11.i.1 See 3.2.b.1
2.11.j Have the child keep a daily writing/reading log. The child writes stories or sentences from which his/her reading lessons can be developed.	2.11.j.1 As reading and writing develop similarly to the language process, by incorporating the child's own language in print, the child learns to read what is most important to him/her. Don't correct the log, but assist the child with consistent errors to correct them himself/herself through a direct teaching task.
2.11.k Provide child with opportunities to expand his/her immediate recall skills.	2.11.k.1 Marston and Larkin (1979) found that an important factor in reading was an opportunity for immediate recall. It made the difference between the achiever and the underachiever.

Techniques for Curriculum Adaptation	Extra Information, Materials or References

3.1 The child has difficulty recalling name of item: will describe it or talk around it, but not recall name.

3.1.a Provide sufficient additional experience both verbally and manipulatively for the child to relate objects and activities to proper terminology.

3.1.a.1 This activity helps develop a phase of language similar to Piaget's Assimilation.

3.1.a.2 For example: when teaching a lesson on fish, utilize a fish tank. Talk about all that is happening in the tank. "The three fishes swim together sometimes and apart at others. Watch the tail fins move through the water. Let's imitate how the tails work with our own hands. Notice how the fishes search the bottom of the tank. What can they be looking for? See how the fish opens his mouth? We learned that was ..." and so on. Provide ample inputs of additional information. Let the children hold a live fish if possible. Use all the senses for input.

3.1.b Expand naming ability through increased exposure to items. Have the child repeat names of objects or pictures of objects. Additional social and language benefits occur when the child practices with a buddy.

3.1.c Provide further experiences with categorization. Go beyond simple categories such as colors and develop more critical discrimination skills such as lightweight circular objects. Let the child experience it through the senses. He/she needs sense interaction in conjunction with verbal interaction.

3.1.c.1 For example: a sensory table might be established. Have items that are circular, oblong, rectangular, cylindrical, etc. in shape. Have the child give as many descriptive words as possible for the items, such as a heavy, rough-edged, long, light yellow piece of wood.

LANGUAGE

Techniques for Curriculum Adaptation	Extra Information, Materials or References

3.1 **The child has difficulty recalling name of item: will describe it or talk around it, but not recall name.** (Continued)

3.1.d Discuss objects or activities in as many different ways as you can devise. Utilize specific vocabulary frequently.

3.1.d.1 Find ways to extend vocabulary usage. Include multiple meanings when child is more advanced.

3.1.d.2 For example: after teaching a lesson about dinosaurs, take some plastic ones and have one child talk or write about what it would be like looking up from a dinosaur's feet and have another child talk or write about what it's like looking down from the head. Mention the specific vocabulary of the name of dinosaur, and the parts of the dinosaur.

3.1.e Delete aspects of the lesson taught when reviewing and have children fit in the necessary pieces.

3.1.f Take a lesson or activity that is well known to the child and break it into parts. Reconstruct the activity. The child will make use of past information to make sense in the present.

3.1.f.1 This activity is working to develop a phase of language acquisition which is similar to Piaget's Accomodation.

3.1.g Reconstruct an entire activity. Use charts or language experience stories to provide a written method for recall.

3.1.g.1 Describe a specific portion of the story or an object and have the child state what part of the story was described or what the name of the object is. You're extending the child's recall and naming capabilities.

3.1.h Small group instruction or one on one instruction will provide more closely monitored input for the child.

Techniques for Curriculum Adaptation	Extra Information, Materials or References

3.1   The child has difficulty recalling name of item: will describe it or talk around it, but not recall name. (Continued)

3.1.i   When a child is floundering and can't find the word, repeat or rephrase, in a positive manner, what he/she is giving you. Also provide additional clues to focus in on the word. Word associations are sometimes helpful.

3.1.i.1   For example: a child can't think of the word 'moon' but tells you it shines in the sky at night and changes shapes throughout the month. An association might be, 'Hey diddle diddle, the cat and the fiddle, the cow jumped over the __?__.'

3.1.i.2   Another word association method would be to give the child several different cues; such as, what is rectangular, soft and your head rests on it?__?__.

3.1.j   If the child repeatedly has difficulty with one particular word, a clue word can be taught to trigger recall of the word with which he or she has difficulty.

3.1.j.1   For example: the child has difficulty recalling the word "horse." When the child is talking and can't think of "horse," the word "neigh" may trigger the word "horse."

3.1.k   Have the child practice describing and naming things as part of class activity. Send a list of difficult words to be practiced at home.

3.1.l   Prepare a log of the difficult words. Include a picture and written description with the name of the item. This log can be used by the child as practice reading material at home.

3.1.m   With young children, further practice on how things are alike and different can be helpful.

LANGUAGE

Techniques for Curriculum Adaptation	Extra Information, Materials or References

3.2   **The child has difficulty with word relationships such as spatial, temporal, or cause and effect.**

3.2.a   Provide ample opportunity to experience and discuss the various relationships. With young children, it is easy to let them get physically involved with activities that include 'first' and 'last.' While involved, talk about who or what is first or last over and over again.

3.2.a.1   'The more hands on activities that can be provided, the more input their memory retrieval system has to pull from to make accurate decisions about incoming messages. The entire time they are experiencing a relationship such as first/last, the verbal input of the other person stating what is happening adds to the language/listening/learning system.

3.2.b   Return to basic classification and categorization activities. For example: with first/last, in a reading lesson group all the words with the first letter 'b' or with the last letter 'n' together. Or group words starting with 'b' that have three letters, etc.

3.2.b.1   Classification and categorization set the groundwork for much of linguistic knowledge. Do everything you can to maximize the acquisition of these skills.

3.2.c   Comment on a child's activities while he or she is doing something. For example: First, Mary pressed the buzzer, the mouse came out of his hole. He ate the cheese. Then, he went back to his hole.

3.2.d   When a child is talking, help by providing a model of appropriate language. This can result in more spontaneous communication but also in better attempts at word usage and comprehension.

3.2.d.1   For example: the child may say: "My doll is seven miles big." The teacher may respond "Wow, you do have a nice seven <u>inch</u> high doll."

Techniques for Curriculum Adaptation	Extra Information, Materials or References

3.2 **The child has difficulty with word relationships such as spatial, temporal, or cause and effect.** (Continued)

3.2.e   Give support cues when possible. For example, if the child is giving a short statement of what happened in the story, the teacher can include the support cues of first/last to help keep him/her on track.

3.2.f   Avoid having the child imitate a response verbally. This only ensures that the child can repeat what was heard. It does not ensure comprehension. When having a child repeat a direction to find miscues, remember that the repetition of the direction only measures memory, not necessarily comprehension of the instruction.

3.3 **The child's conversations jump through different topics within one conversation.**

3.3.a   Keep your language simple.

3.3.a.1   If the language structures of sentences are too complex, the child will stop listening to what is being said and go off on a tangent.

3.3.a.2   The child may misunderstand a word or idea in the conversation. That misunderstood word leads his/her train of thought to what seems like a new idea to the teacher but for the child, is continuous.

3.3.a.3   The child is often unaware of the effect of his/her scattered conversation to the listener because the conversation followed what seemed a logical progression to him/her.

LANGUAGE

Techniques for Curriculum Adaptation	Extra Information, Materials or References

3.3   The child's conversations jump through different topics within one conversation. (Continued)

3.3.b   Try to evaluate how the conversation changed. Did the child misconstrue a word? What word did he/she hear incorrectly? When the child is older, it helps to point out the possible misrepresentation of words.

3.3.b.1   For example: the conversation may have been talking about the amount of "hits" in a baseball game. The child may start talking about the "ships" in the "bay." This sounds totally out of sync with the rest of the conversation but the child could have heard "hits" as "ships" and "game" as "bay." He/she did not focus in on the rest of the linguistic message and proceeded off on his/her own tangent.

3.3.c   Provide the child with organizational models of time structure.

3.3.c.1   The child may not be internally organized to be able to keep to one task for any length of time. Structure the routine in the rest of the child's day so that his/her world makes sense. This structure may eventually carry over into conversational skills.

3.3.c.2   For example: keep the same schedule every day when possible. Talk your way from activity to activity. When one activity ends, tell the children what will be next before having them move to that activity. This might seem overly simple, but it develops time and actitivy sequencing skills.

3.3.d   Provide activities in pragmatics. Help them understand the effects of communication behaviors on other participants. Pragmatics refers to the cause and effect of the child's communication behavior.

3.3.d.1   This deals with the relationship level of communication. Many young otitis media affected children do not understand this level and need more experience with it. (Hubbell, 1977)

3.3.d.2   For example: when a child repeatedly shouts out answers, discuss how this affects the other children around

Techniques for Curriculum Adaptation	Extra Information, Materials or References

3.3 The child's conversations jump through different topics within one conversation. (Continued)

		him/her. This should be done privately, so as not to diminish his/her self-esteem.
3.3.e	Ensure that the acoustics of the room are appropriate.	3.3.e.1 This will prevent sounds being masked by extraneous noise and will provide maximum opportunity for listening.
3.3.f	Be aware that the child may not have the language skills to continue with the discussion as started. His/her thoughts are more comfortable elsewhere. He/she directs everyone's attention there.	3.3.f.1 For example: the activity may involve a series of four activities or ideas. The child may only be able to handle three, so starts to talk about a totally different subject because what the teacher was doing became too difficult.
3.3.g	Amplify your voice. This may provide the extra input needed to ensure maximum listening and comprehension. The child will make fewer jumps if he/she is processing information adequately.	3.3.g.1 Sound field amplification and sound enhancement systems may be helpful.

3.4 The child answers questions inappropriately.

3.4.a	Evaluate the question form used and the language contained within it.	3.4.a.1 Children may have confusion with word relationships, ie. spatial (first/last), temporal (before/after), and cause and effect statements (if, then). Think about the inappropriate response in relation to the words in the question.
		3.4.a.2 The otitis media affected child may have difficulty with plurals, possessives, and regular past tenses.

LANGUAGE

Techniques for Curriculum Adaptation	Extra Information, Materials or References

3.4   The child answers questions inappropriately. (Continued)

	3.4.a.3 The child may have difficulty with irregular verb tenses, noun plurals and with verbs where the vowel changes from the present to past tense (run to ran). Consider all the parts of the language used.
	3.4.a.4 The child may have difficulty with modal verbs (may, might, must, should), auxiliary verbs (has, have, is, are), prepositions and articles.
	3.4.a.5 The child may misinterpret the passive voice, conjunctions, and negations.
	3.4.a.6 The child may interpret literally what is meant to be abstract or figurative language.
3.4.b Provide opportunities to discuss clarification strategies.	3.4.b.1 The child may not feel comfortable enough with his/her input and output retrieval systems to ask for further clarification. He/she then may respond with an answer which might fit the question as he/she interpreted it.
	3.4.b.2 For example: when a child follows through on an aural direction incorrectly, talk to him/her privately. Ask him/her to tell you what the direction was. Evaluate what the child said and try to find out where the breakdown took place. Then go through the direction again. Use simple language in smaller steps. By talking with the child, you can understand how the child heard the direction. Be sure to make the child feel he/she is not being

Techniques for Curriculum Adaptation	Extra Information, Materials or References

3.4   The child answers questions inappropriately. (Continued)

punished but that you're glad you were able to work together.

3.4.c Ensure a proper acoustic environment.

3.4.c.1 Provide every opportunity to maximize the input message. By limiting extraneous noise, more of the input message can be received with which to formulate a more appropriate answer.

3.4.d Provide opportunities for open discussion versus direct questioning.

3.4.d.1 Open discussion has less verbal structure. The child can take what he/she needs from the discussion and can use as much of it as necessary to understand. Direct questioning limits input and comprehension abilities.

3.4.e Restructure the prosody, intonation and emphasis of the question asked.

3.4.e.1 Children often take a long time to answer questions or answer inappropriately because they have failed to understand the question. Prosody, intonation and emphasis are what give meaning to most sentences. Adjust how you say questions by varying these three areas and better comprehension may result.

3.5   The child has difficulty waiting for his/her turn.

3.5.a Impart to the child that what he/she says is important and that he/she will be called on.

3.5.a.1 This message can be passed on through a wink, a finger raised indicating "Just one minute," or simple verbal interaction discussing the issue with the child.

LANGUAGE

Techniques for Curriculum Adaptation	Extra Information, Materials or References

3.5   The child has difficulty waiting for his/her turn. (Continued)

	3.5.a.2 Frequently, the child has had difficulty putting his/her thoughts together. He/she is proud of that thought and wants to share this accomplishment with others. The child may also be afraid that he/she will forget the message so wants to say it before he/she forgets.
3.5.b Provide opportunities to discuss the pragmatics of language. Help the child understand the effects of his/her communication behaviors on others. Pragmatics refers to the cause and effect of the child's communication behavior.	3.5.b.1 The child may not realize how his/her lack of turn-taking skills affects others. He/she may not be able to stop his/her impulsivity, but an awareness of proper roles will help.
	3.5.b.2 With older children, a videotape can allow the children to view their interaction skills. The class can critique and discuss ways to improve or change.
	3.5.b.3 Discuss turn taking protocols. Develop more appropriate formats.
	3.5.b.4 For example: the child may constantly interrupt you while you are talking to someone else. In private, discuss how this is considered an inappropriate behavior and tell the child how this makes you feel. The child may not be able to control his/her impulsivity. But through understanding and guidance, you can help the child learn how the improper use of language affects others in social situations.

Techniques for Curriculum Adaptation	Extra Information, Materials or References

3.5 The child has difficulty waiting for his/her turn. (Continued)

		3.5.b.5	For example: a child did something wrong and smiled up at the teacher. To many people, this may "show that the child did it on purpose." In reality, the child smiled because he/she didn't know how else to act. Discuss the outcome of smiling versus other appropriate behaviors.
3.5.c	Provide opportunities for the child to respond quickly as well as not so quickly.	3.5.c.1	The child's internal system for information needs to be extended. The child may feel uncomfortable responding to questions; or may have difficulty formulating a response. He/she wants to share it and get positive feedback. If the child is reinforced by being called on quickly, the degree can be extended by ensuring him/her an opportunity to respond every time he/she raises his/her hand. (Within the limits of the situations, of course). The child needs to experience positive reactions in order to stretch his/her delay gratification time.

3.6 The child may use a rehearsed phrase to mean many things ("too big" may mean "too large, " "too many", etc.)

3.6.a	Provide opportunities to expand vocabulary.	3.6.a.1	Frequently, the child has had success sharing his/her thoughts by using the rehearsed phrase. He/she may not know the correct word for the situation he/she is in, but the other word had been successful before, and it covers the main thought. So the child will use it to share his/her ideas successfully again.

LANGUAGE

Techniques for Curriculum Adaptation	Extra Information, Materials or References

3.6 The child may use a rehearsed phrase to mean many things ("too big" may mean "too large, " "too many", etc.) (Continued)

3.6.b   Provide appropriate language modeling.

3.6.b.1   Teachers can comment on the child's activities, expand utterances, or discuss a shared experience.

3.6.b.2   For example: while the child is playing, talk about what he/she is doing. "The ball rolls up. The ball rolls down. Now, you can bounce the ball."

3.6.b.3   For example: the child says, "See my new ball." The teacher responds, "Yes, I see your new green-striped ball. I like it."

3.6.c   Repeat the phrase as the child has said it and then expand upon it. For example: "Yes, that ladder is too big. It is very large. It is a very tall, high ladder."

3.7 The child has difficulty predicting story outcomes.

3.7.a   Provide opportunities to visually represent the story line with activities, pictures, slides, or a movie. Before reaching the conclusion, create possible outcomes by thinking, and then by doing further activities.

3.7.a.1   With a movie or videotape, stop before the end, discuss outcomes, then see the ending. Later discuss why and how the ending occurred.

Techniques for Curriculum Adaptation	Extra Information, Materials or References

3.7   The child has difficulty predicting story outcomes. (Continued)

3.7.b   Prepare stories with three simple parts before dealing with more involved stories.

3.7.b.1   Go over the first two parts and have the child guess what can happen next before going to the third part. As "hands-on" experience is helpful, do stories that can be physically enacted. For example: get an object to represent a present, then bring out the wrapping paper and ribbon; discuss what will happen next before wrapping the present.

3.7.c   Discuss classroom activities during and after they happen.

3.7.c.1   Put up a sequence chart of up to five sections. Then, as class activities are done, jot down briefly the substeps for each activity. For example: After the morning exercises where the teacher discusses or says what is coming next, break down the parts into substeps. Substep 1, Mary took attendance; Substep 2, John led the pledge of allegiance, etc.

3.7.c.2   The otitis media affected children function best with order in their lives. Provide consistent activities for them so that they are able to predict usual outcomes to their daily lives. Build upon the consistent activities in a story form.

3.7.d   Provide more language input. Talk about what you're doing as you are doing it. Rephrase and repeat frequently.

3.7.d.1   The child may simply not have experienced a similar episode in his/her life from which to draw a conclusion to the present activity. Talking about everything as it is being done or experienced can provide the language for the child to store and retrieve at a later time.

3.7.d.2   Instead of demanding or expecting the story outcome from a child with

LANGUAGE

Techniques for Curriculum Adaptation	Extra Information, Materials or References
3.7 The child has difficulty predicting story outcomes. (Continued)	
	weaknesses in this area, provide the child with the language necessary for the story's end but also go beyond and explain the ending in detail.
3.7.e Create a "could this have happened" game.	**3.7.e.1** Make up stories that are either real or far-fetched. Discuss with the children the difference between the two. Emphasize the why's. The otitis media affected child often is very literal and more needs to be done to overcome this weakness.
	3.7.e.2 Have children create silly or real stories and discuss why each story could be real or not.
3.7.f First read well-known stories and discuss outcomes. Then relate to new ones that either the children make up or that are in the literature.	**3.7.f.1** Suggest to parents that they can help children find or draw pictures to put stories together. The visual representations often allow the children to understand things that they may not have understood otherwise.

3.8   **The child has difficulty with plurals, possessives, and irregular past tenses.**

3.8.a   Provide an appropriate acoustic environment such as with sound field amplification or sound enhancement systems.

3.8.a.1   During early development, the child may have missed subtle auditory cues. Cues that provide stress changes, inflections, pitch, loudness, rhythm, duration, and timbre may have been processed inaccurately and learned inaccurately. The child doesn't have the correct forms stored and learned in his/her memory. With an appropriate acoustical environment, the child can receive the correct cues; however, the old ways have to be "unlearned."

3.8.a.2   Make sure distractions are at a minimum. The child will perceive the correct form much easier and quicker if he/she is hearing the sound appropriately. The Sound Enhancement System allows for direct teacher input to the child's ear. Therefore, the child may not continue with incorrect language forms.

3.8.b   Avoid correcting the child's errors. Instead, repeat what the child has said utilizing the correct grammatical form.

3.8.b.1   Frequently, as children mature, and the correct forms are emphasized by the speakers around them, their ears begin to notice a difference between what they are saying and what they are hearing. If the change is self-motivated, then the children retain a good feeling of self-worth because they are the ones making the change – it is not being demanded of them.

LANGUAGE

Techniques for Curriculum Adaptation	Extra Information, Materials or References

3.8   The child has difficulty with plurals, possessives, and irregular past tenses. (Continued)

3.8.c   In a one-on-one lesson or small group instruction, have the child repeat the correct form after the instructor.

3.8.c.1   This should be done in a situation where others are being given the same instruction. A whole lesson can be extended to include the verb tense, plural form, etc. that needs to be taught. For example: a lesson about birds can be extended to teach "went" instead of "goed." As the teacher talks about the flight path of birds, "went" can be used and emphasized frequently. All the children can be made to repeat the sentence with the correct verb in it.

3.8.d   Discuss appropriate techniques for individualized problems with the speech/language pathologist.

3.8.e   Make sure that the child maintains eye contact during instructions.

3.8.e.1   Sometimes the visual sense can be more sensitive than the auditory sense. By maintaining eye contact, the children focus attention more directly on what is being said.

3.8.e.2   For the child whose self-concept is very weak, this activity may be too frustrating. The stress of watching while being uncomfortable can negate the advantage of the visual sense.

Techniques for Curriculum Adaptation	Extra Information, Materials or References

3.9   The child is very literal.

3.9.a   Provide opportunity for explanations for what might be the simplest of statements. For example: If discussing a race and the phrase "the heat is on" is used, the child may envision a race track being excessively hot.

3.9.a.1   Jokes or idioms are often not understood by this child. As the child was learning language, he/she made sense to his/her world of fluctuating limited sound by making use of everything that was organized and structured. The subtleties of language were often missed and, therefore, the child learned 'literal' language. As the child matures, the 'abstract' language cues, idioms, figures of speech, etc. must be explained.

3.9.b   Prepare a list of idioms. Explain each one and have all the children draw pictures or write a paragraph of the incorrect meaning and then the correct meaning. For example: it's raining cats and dogs." Children frequently picture dogs and cats falling out of the sky. Explain the correct meaning.

3.9.b.1   Most otitis media affected children must be specifically taught each idiom. It's best to introduce the idioms indirectly through various lessons whenever appropriate.

3.9.b.2   Open discussion works best for comprehension. The child is not put on the spot for not comprehending and can absorb input from the discussion.

3.9.b.3   Prepare pictures of the idioms whenever possible. The child will be better able to remember the idiom's meaning when provided with many different input modes.

3.9.b.4   Go over the list day after day to ensure comprehension. Try to continue this activity throughout the entire year, not just one portion of a year. Language comprehension is ongoing.

LANGUAGE

Techniques for Curriculum Adaptation	Extra Information, Materials or References
3.9 **The child is very literal.** (Continued)	
3.9.c Create opportunities to discuss real and make-believe stories.	3.9.c.1 Make-believe can be a difficult concept for the otitis media affected child. Frequently, fairy tales and cartoons are believed as real. As with idioms, the child needs frequent opportunities to discuss real versus non-real.
	3.9.c.2 Involve the parents by having them read fairy tales to the children and then discuss why they are not real.
3.9.d Create opportunities to discuss fact versus opinion.	3.9.d.1 This would be especially beneficial for the older child who can understand more of the other complexities of language.
	3.9.d.2 Make a fact versus opinion chart. During open conversations, children's arguments, television commercials, etc., plot the difference between fact versus opinion. Always include explanations.
3.9.e If, after restating the phrase, a child responds with a blank expression on his/her face, rephrase what was said.	3.9.e.1 Perhaps the statement was heard but did not make sense to the child. The rephrasing provides another way for the child to comprehend.
3.9.f Provide opportunities in one-on-one situations to allow the child to explain what he/she thought was said.	3.9.f.1 This technique often provides the teacher with a better understanding of the child and allows him/her to clarify misconceptions.
	3.9.f.2 This technique should not be utilized with large groups because the child 1) may not feel comfortable explaining what was heard, 2) may not know the words needed to explain the sentence and 3) may be turned off to wanting to respond later.

Techniques for Curriculum Adaptation	Extra Information, Materials or References

3.9   The child is very literal. (Continued)

3.9.g	Increase child's exposure to non-literal ideas. For example: "the leaves whistled in the breeze" is a sentence in which the child may picture leaves whistling.	3.9.g.1	Try to create activities that fit into your regular curriculum that may be able to teach an idiom, for example. Science, social studies, and reading activities are good for this.
3.9.h	Comment on activity or lesson as it is happening. Whenever possible, say each new thought two or three different ways.	3.9.h.1	For example: A discussion around Christopher Columbus may include: "He sailed the Seven Seas. He followed the ocean blue." The literal child may actually see seven little seas with blue lines spread throughout and connecting them. This lesson could be used to explain these meanings.

3.10   The child uses inappropriate pronoun references. Example: may start with one form and then change the form later.

3.10.a	Support cues are helpful.	3.10.a.1	The child may use different pronouns within one sentence for the same person. As the teacher, respond afterward with a rephrasing of the sentence but verbally emphasizing, with a slightly raised voice, the corrected form. For example, Child: "He ran down the street and when she saw the dog, he ran back home." Teacher: "So, when he saw the dog, he ran home. I guess _he_ was afraid.
3.10.b	Reinforce pronoun usage with picture clues.	3.10.b.1	Make a chart of the words with pictures and refer to the chart frequently in discussions.

LANGUAGE

Techniques for Curriculum Adaptation	Extra Information, Materials or References
3.10 **The child uses inappropriate pronoun references.** Example: may start with one form and then change the form later. (Continued)	
3.10.c Find stories with one boy, one girl or with boys and girls. Have the child relate the story using only pronouns.	3.10.c.1 As the child is relating the story, pictures can be used to reinforce the correct usage. Have the child double check his/her responses by seeing if, indeed, the girl or boy did what was indicated.
3.10.d When reading a story, use Sound Field Amplification and emphasize correct pronouns.	3.10.d.1 The story telling (with pictures when possible) is an enjoyable way to learn. The extra loudness from the amplification can stimulate the brain to receive the needed lesson of pronoun comprehension and perhaps, usage.
3.10.e Sound Enhancement Systems can provide direct auditory input and enable the child to hear the difference between the emphasized pronouns.	3.10.e.1 By stimulating and emphasizing the words with the direct input, the child may be able to receive the information better.
3.10.f Have the children create a song using the correct pronoun form with puppets for visual reinforcement.	3.10.f.1 A simple song such as "He, he, he, he, she; she, she, she, she, he; These are two people you see; So make sure if it's he or she," can be used. Hold two simple boy and girl puppets in hand while singing the song and emphasize the correct one when the pronoun is said.
	3.10.f.2 Transfer the idea of song and puppet to sentences. Have the puppet be the carry-over as a visual reinforcement to stress correct pronoun usage.

Techniques for Curriculum Adaptation	Extra Information, Materials or References

3.11   The child has difficulty extracting the main idea of a paragraph or story.

3.11.a   Ensure appropriate acoustic environment.

3.11.a.1   Use sound field amplification, sound enhancement system, or personal amplification to ensure that the child is getting appropriate input without background distractions.

3.11.b   When possible, emphasize the main idea by raising the volume of your voice. Allow the child to hear the important part a little bit louder than the rest of the paragraph or story.

3.11.b.1   The increased volume singles out what is important and triggers the auditory nerve even more so than usual.

3.11.c   Have the child repeat the parts of the paragraph that he/she remembers. Ask him what is important/not important. Ask the child to identify various key items. Do this without judgment in actions or tone of voice.

3.11.c.1   This method allows the teacher to understand a little bit better how the child puts the language he/she is hearing to use. Being non-judgmental in your response is critical because the child needs to feel good about his/her open responses.

3.11.c.2   From this breakdown, one should begin to see what the child responds to and perhaps gear the child to listen for other specific items.

3.11.c.3   This technique also allows the teacher to evaluate if the language used in the paragraph was too difficult for the child.

3.11.c.4   It is important not to second guess the child. Sometimes, the language problems are so subtle that the child may understand much of what was said and only not comprehend a small portion of what was heard. However, that small portion may be what leads to the confusion.

LANGUAGE

Techniques for Curriculum Adaptation	Extra Information, Materials or References

3.11 **The child has difficulty extracting the main idea of a paragraph or story. (Continued)**

3.11.d   Break down the parts of the paragraph or story using visual representations whenever possible.

3.11.d.1   The visual reinforcement may trigger a comprehension of the whole that might not have taken place otherwise.

3.11.d.2   For example: when reading a folk tale which does not include a picture book, such as <u>The Elves and the Shoemaker</u>, provide either extra pictures or visual actions to reinforce the parts of the story.

3.11.e   Teach the child to visualize auditory input.

3.11.e.1   Begin with simple activities such as letters and numbers, then proceed to sentences. Have the child form a picture in his/her mind of what is being described. Build upon this skill over time.

3.11.e.2   When a skill is learned, have the child visualize the paragraph or story. Then ask what was the most important or the main idea. Making a visual representation often allows the child to bring clarity to what was said.

3.12 **The child has difficulty putting his/her thoughts into words.**

3.12.a   First and foremost, try to understand the child's frustration.

3.12.a.1   Allow the child's tears to come. Perhaps the frustration comes out in the form of stomping feet or whininess. Perhaps the child has learned to rebel as a way to avoid this kind of difficult situation.

Techniques for Curriculum Adaptation	Extra Information, Materials or References

3.12   The child has difficulty putting his/her thoughts into words. (Continued)

3.12.a.2 Until the child knows that you will try to understand him/her, the behaviors will continue and perhaps increase. Whenever possible, they should be tolerated until a behavior modification program can be implemented. Behavior modification is only suggested when the child's problems are understood because if the pressure the child is experiencing is not diminished, the behavior modification will only create greater inner frustration and diminish his/her struggling self-esteem.

3.12.b Supply helping words at times, being sure to praise the contribution of any correct or useful ideas the child gives.

3.12.b.1 Supplying too many words can be detrimental. The child needs to feel as though he/she was able to relate the idea of the sentence.

3.12.c When the child is having difficulty retrieving a word, but the rest of the idea is present, supplying the word is helpful.

3.12.c.1 Sometimes, you will find a child with significant word retrieval problems. Providing useful, contextual examples or opportunities to try words is helpful as long as the word will be provided when the child is unable to produce it.

3.12.c.2 The child often knows the word/words, that he/she wants to use, but can't recall it from memory . This creates frustration which can be diminished by using creative ways to recall it. Frequently, teachers comment that the child talks around the word. The teacher can, in turn, provide the clues "around" the item to get the child to recall the word. For example: the child is having difficulty remembering the name of the 'sun' but can tell you all about it.

LANGUAGE

Techniques for Curriculum Adaptation	Extra Information, Materials or References

3.12 **The child has difficulty putting his/her thoughts into words.** (Continued)

So the teacher uses all the descriptive words such as, It's round. It shines during the day. It gives us heat. The thing that shines during the day is the _____." Sometimes, when presented in this way, the child will remember the word, but not when asked directly.

3.12.d Allow the child plenty of time to express his/her thoughts without making him/her uncomfortable.

3.12.e In a one-on-one situation, help the child break down his/her thoughts into simpler structures. By having less to put together, some children can remember the word.

3.12.e.1 For example: the child has difficulty giving the answer to a question. The answer to the question, "What is the boy doing?" may be too difficult. Break the picture down in parts. "I see a boy. Here is a bike. Is the boy on the bike? What does he do with the bike?"

3.12.e.2 For example: the child is told to draw a red circle between two bears. He/she doesn't know what to do. The child knows "between" and "circle" and "bears," but can't put them together. Take each part and demonstrate separately. Then work to get the child to comprehend the meaning of the instruction in combination.

Techniques for Curriculum Adaptation	Extra Information, Materials or References

4.1 The child exhibits overactivity: he/she uses it as a means of investigation, goal fulfillment or method of communication. The actions are often purposeful.

4.1.a Develop activities where the child can become physically involved. Hands on activities will stimulate the other senses and enhance learning.

4.1.a.1 Use as many physical objects as possible to provide visual cues.

4.1.a.2 Know that the child needs to react by touching others or manipulating objects and make allowances. Find a child for the otitis media affected child to sit next to who doesn't mind being physically invaded.

In other words, some children do not mind being touched or being in close proximity to other people, while some children mind very much. Of course, the child chosen should not trigger an increase in the otitis media affected child's overactive behavior.

4.1.a.3 In a group discussion or teacher lecture, allow the child to sit in an area where his/her physical movement won't be disruptive, e.g. on the very edge or back of the group, or on the side in the front, which ever is least distracting to the teacher and other students.

4.1.a.4 The child often needs to move his/her body when an activity is auditorily or linguistically taxing. If the child is forced to remain still, he/she places all his/her energy and efforts into being still, and the activity is put on the back burner. This is especially true when the child is trying to listen. He or she may need to wriggle or squirm to adequately process the auditory message.

SOCIALIZATION

Techniques for Curriculum Adaptation	Extra Information, Materials or References

4.1   The child exhibits overactivity: he/she uses it as a means of investigation, goal fulfillment or method of communication. The actions are often purposeful. (Continued)

4.1.b Take away some of the stimuli being presented. Keep the physical presence of objects to a minimum.	
4.1.c Use as many visual or tactile cues as possible to enhance the presentation.	
4.1.d Instead of simply talking, gesture or demonstrate as an alternative means of learning.	
4.1.e Try not to overtax the child's capabilities. i.e. try to use language that is simple and direct; keep sequential activities to a minimum; interject visual reinforcement when possible.	
4.1.f Teach the learning task in simple, direct phrases and then rephrase and repeat it.	4.1.f.1 For example: when introducing a lesson on size, use simple direct phrases. "The elephant is big. The goat is small." Rephrase: "The elephant is very large. The goat next to the elephant is little." Repeat: "The elephant is big. The goat is small."
4.1.g Ensure a proper acoustical environment. Extraneous noises will over tax their sense system.	4.1.g.1 The make-up of the room, the positioning of objects, and the addition of sound absorbing materials is very important in controlling the acoustics. The use of carpeting, curtains, bookcases and other large objects can do much to cut down on reverberation. For further sources on classroom acoustics, consult Berg (1987) and Ross (1972).

Techniques for Curriculum Adaptation	Extra Information, Materials or References

4.1 The child exhibits overactivity: he/she uses it as a means of investigation, goal fulfillment or method of communication. The actions are often purposeful. (Continued)

4.1.h Child needs goal directional tasks (build in complexity but start with simple tasks); ie: tasks which will produce a desired outcome. An example would be, "John will sit with the group and will touch his neighbor no more than three times."

4.1.h.1 The child may actually be unsure if he/she should be listening for enjoyment, for comprehension or for directional tasks. With young children, you may want to use a chart indicating which listening task is at hand. Example: Label the top of the chart with the listening tasks and then place a big circle around the one which is occurring.

4.1.h.2 Go over examples of what a directional task might be. Later, after giving a direction, have the class vote on whether it was a direction. For example: the teacher says, "Everyone sit down and take out your workbooks." The children decide if it is a direction.

4.1.h.3 To avoid singling out the otitis media affected child and placing him/her in a stressful situation, work out a behavioral interaction with the child. After giving a direction, nod or wink to the child to ensure that he/she knows a direction is given. After a number of good responses, have him/her try it alone and reward him/her positively when he/she does.

4.1.h.4 Role playing is a good tool to use to teach a child the differentiation between a statement of fact and direction.

SOCIALIZATION

Techniques for Curriculum Adaptation	Extra Information, Materials or References

4.1   **The child exhibits overactivity: he/she uses it as a means of investigation, goal fulfillment or method of communication. The actions are often purposeful.** (Continued)

	4.1.h.5 Utilizing the directions for making phone calls is a fun way to distinguish between statement and direction.

4.2   **The child is distractible: other senses interfere with the ability to concentrate on a task.**

4.2.a Arrange seat work so that it is to be done at a single desk, not a table. Place the desk in a location with few visual distractions such as books, objects, people moving, etc. and few auditory distractions, such as fan motor noises or people talking.	4.2.a.1 A portable carrel can sometimes be very helpful in blocking out visual distractions.
	4.2.a.2 Use earmuffs to block out extraneous auditory distractions.
	4.2.a.3 Some children work well independently when you allow music to be played via a walkman radio or tape player. The music stimulates a different center in the brain and may counteract the verbal background noise. However, whatever is allowed for one child, must be allowed for the other children, whether it be music, earmuffs or the use of a carrel.
4.2.b Use physical closeness or a hand-on-the-shoulder to draw attention to the fact that a subject is being discussed to which the child needs to listen.	4.2.b.1 In group situations, input may overtax their systems and result in improper behaviors. Allowances should be made for their inability to control their actions at the time.
	4.2.b.2 See other suggestions under 4.1.h.1, 4.1.h.2 and 4.1.h.3.

Techniques for Curriculum Adaptation	Extra Information, Materials or References

4.2 **The child is distractible: other senses interfere with the ability to concentrate on a task.** (Continued)

4.2.c   Use a positive response to the negative situation. For example, say "You have your pencil ready to work." Never mind that the child is sprawled across the desk or staring out the window.

4.2.c.1   This is a behavioral modification technique in which you comment only on the positive. "Catch them doing something right", and comment on that!

4.2.d   Use the child's name in a statement as a way to pull him/her back into the situation. "John/Jane, you have your pencil ready to work."

4.2.e   In small or large group teaching situations, sound field amplification emphasizes the teacher's voice and this input may override the other distracting inputs.

4.2.e.1   For sources of sound field amplification apparatus, see the Appendix.

4.2.f   Emphasize key words by slightly raising the intensity of the voice, thereby stimulating the auditory input.

Techniques for Curriculum Adaptation	Extra Information, Materials or References

4.3 The child does not participate in class, but when he/she does, may give an inappropriate response.

4.3.a Teacher should listen to what the child's response is and try to incorporate it if possible. At the same time, try to evaluate what he/she might have been processing. Perhaps the words he/she thought were said were nothing like what was actually said.

4.3.a.1 For example, the teacher might have been talking about a 'house.' The child may have only heard the 'ow' sound and not processed the /h/ and /s/ and then thought the conversation was about a "cow." This answer would be very far fetched indeed. The child may have had similar confusions in the rest of the words used in the discussion. Sometimes, the child does not hear or attend to all the words being said. He/she may only focus in on key words which, if heard incorrectly, would greatly alter the ability to interact appropriately in a discussion.

4.3.a.2 Try, if possible, to incorporate the child's idea so that he/she will not feel embarrassed. Participation needs to be encouraged. As long as the child's self-esteem remains positive, interaction, even though inappropriate, may continue.

4.3.a.3 An Educational Audiologist may want to look at specific speech sounds in noise when testing the child and perform a phoneme analysis for a clearer picture of the child's problem sound errors.

4.3.a.4 The child may have poor auditory discrimination for social discourse in a noisy listening environment.

Techniques for Curriculum Adaptation	Extra Information, Materials or References

4.3   The child does not participate in class, but when he/she does, may give an inappropriate response. (Continued)

4.3.b   Sound field amplification will raise the teacher's voice intensity sufficiently and thus allow the child to hear all the sounds of the conversation accurately.

           4.3.b.1   See 2.5.e.1

4.3.c   Personal sound amplification can be useful in both small and large group discussions as a means to subdue the extraneous noises.

           4.3.c.1   See 2.5.e.1

4.3.d   A sound enhancement system might be useful in a small to large group situation because it blocks out much of the extraneous noise.

           4.3.d.1   See 2.5.e.1

4.3.e   Include as many visual devices for the lesson being taught without making them overwhelming. Introduce the items one at a time. The new items should not get in the way of the ones presented. Extraneous visual objects in the room should be limited when introducing something new.

4.3.f   Try to position yourself close to the child during discussions or presentations. The physical closeness often triggers the child to attend.

4.3.g   Make sure the children are aware that a listening task is at hand. Often they hear sound and don't use it so they don't know that they should be listening. Work out a signal for them to be aware that they should be listening.

           4.3.g.1   Inconsistent sensory input during the formative years may lead children to ignore or block sensory input at times. (Howie, 1975)

SOCIALIZATION

Techniques for Curriculum Adaptation	Extra Information, Materials or References

4.4 **The child manipulates objects or uses class materials inappropriately** (bangs pencil on the desk, stares at a pencil on the desk while the teacher is talking, places body physically away from the teacher, such as turning sideways on the chair).

4.4.a With an older child, discuss what he/she is doing and try to work through more appropriate strategies for him/her to use in coping with a situation.	4.4.a.1 The kinesthetic/tactile response is probably more acute in some otitis media affected children because when sensory input was developing in infancy, the auditory deprivation forced these other senses to develop more finely.
	4.4.a.2 The child often is not doing this to be stubborn, or rude, but is working out his/her frustration or anxiety over the task at hand. He/she is often unaware of what is happening. Internally, the child is aware that something is too taxing. It could be the language the teacher is using, the difficulty of the task at hand, the rate of the teacher's speech, or the level of background noise.
4.4.b Avoid taking the object away from the child if at all possible.	4.4.b.1 Any learning that the teacher hoped to accomplish is often eliminated when the child's world is altered. By taking the object away or enforcing a different behavior, you have altered the child's internal world. This may cause more difficulty because the child can't function with that change.
4.4.c If the activity is not disrupting or interrupting the classroom activity, it is beneficial to ignore the act or bring the child into a different activity.	4.4.c.1 It's like trying to get the active child to sit still. All their energy goes into sitting still and learning can't occur.

Techniques for Curriculum Adaptation	Extra Information, Materials or References

4.5   The child is prone to tantrums.

4.5.a   Ignore the tantrum.

4.5.a.1   Although the tantrum comes out of total frustration from some experience, the response is learned. Once the child learns that the tantrum has not accomplished its purpose, then more appropriate behaviors can be tried and encouraged.

4.5.b   If necessary, remove the child from the classroom if he/she is disturbing others and then ignore the tantrum. Of course, the child should remain supervised.

4.5.b.1   Try to understand the causative factors of the tantrums. If possible, try to alter the rate of speech, desired tasks, level of noise, etc. to decrease the likelihood of improper responses in the future.

4.5.c   Offer praise to the child when something occurs which may have caused a tantrum in the past but the child managed to control it.

4.5.c.1   The child needs reinforcement that he/she is a good person and that you still care.

4.6   The child withdraws from classroom activity (also includes the category of daydreaming).

4.6.a   Change presentation modes. Try a few different ways to see if the child will attend any better.

4.6.a.1   For example, try having objects for the child to touch and see, auditory discourse, slide or filmstrips, VCR, hands-on making something. Change or alter throughout to keep the child's attention.

4.6.b   Sound field amplification is a way to amplify the teacher's voice over the entire classroom. It may provide just enough extra input for the child to receive the message auditorily.

4.6.b.1   See 2.5.e.1.

SOCIALIZATION

Techniques for Curriculum Adaptation	Extra Information, Materials or References
4.6 **The child withdraws from classroom activity** (also includes the category of daydreaming). (Continued)	
4.6.c Personal sound amplification can be used for small group instruction.	4.6.c.1 See 2.5.e.1.
	4.6.c.2 Sometimes the child's senses simply need to be stimulated the slightest bit more in order to get his/her attention. Slight forms of amplification can accomplish this.
4.6.d Where extraneous background noise is troublesome, a sound enhancement system is beneficial.	4.6.d.1 See 2.5.e.1
	4.6.d.2 By getting the teacher's or other children's direct input, the child is stimulating the auditory pathway directly. The child often does not withdraw as frequently or at all when the input signal is sufficient but not overdone.
4.6.e Avoid over taxing the body's listening and learning requirements.	4.6.e.1 Sometimes the children simply need to engage in physically involved free play as a means of getting rid of frustrations and permitting them to continue afterwards. Their bodies need a break from one kind of task.
4.7 **The child prefers to be alone or removed when the noise levels get too much.**	
4.7.a Have a corner or place in the classroom which all children can use as a time-out space.	4.7.a.1 Some children's systems reach saturation. To avoid inappropriate behavior, they need to monitor their responses. If they feel that they can't handle things, the time-out space gives them a spot to escape to. It should be discussed that they use the time not for play time but for a "time alone" time.

Techniques for Curriculum Adaptation	Extra Information, Materials or References

4.7 **The child prefers to be alone or removed when the noise levels get too much.** (Continued)

4.7.b	The Sound Enhancement system can be set to provide only teacher-directed input.	4.7.b.1	This teacher only input can be helpful when the noise in the background is too great. Amplifying only the teacher helps block out the noises.
4.7.c.	The child might be encouraged to try earmuffs if the activity is a self-directed or at the desk activity.	4.7.c.1	In order to reduce extraneous noise, earmuffs reduce the amount of noise in the background.

4.8 **The child likes to be read to.**

4.8.	Encourage classmates or siblings who can read fluently to read to the child.	4.8.a.1	Although this isn't an actual "problem," it is one descriptor of the otitis media affected child. The child may have frustrations because he/she isn't able to read by himself/herself. By continuing the enjoyment and pleasure of the voice with its language, the child is still kept interested in learning.
		4.8.a.2	Some young children who are just learning to read may distort the flow of the story sufficiently enough that the otitis media affected child doesn't want that child to read to him/her. The beginning reader who has to sound out words and reads each word separately, alters the rhythm, inflections, frequency characteristics, stress patterns and timing of both the words themselves and the sentence. This makes comprehension almost impossible for the otitis media affected child who needs to hear normal language. It's like hearing a foreign language to the child.

SOCIALIZATION

Techniques for Curriculum Adaptation	Extra Information, Materials or References

4.9   **The child is often unaware of the needs of others** (also the intentions of others).

4.9.a The child needs more exposure to categorization and classification of sounds of others – the vocal cues of discomfort or actual body movement sounds.	**4.9.a.1** Very often the child does not have the linguistic capabilities to understand the subtle messages received.
	4.9.a.2 The child may have difficulty determining the subtleties of the voice in stress patterns – the inflections, sarcasm, anger, disbelief (Skinner, 1978). The child's responses may be inconsistent.
4.9.b Explain the pragmatics of interpersonal communication, ie: the effects of how they say things to others, how they behave when they are talking and when others are talking, or the impressions others perceive of them in any interaction.	**4.9.b.1** Very often the child is not aware of the effects his/her communication behavior has on the other participant and vice versa. (Hubbell, 1977)
	4.9.b.2 For example: plan a lesson about how people act in a group, when others are talking, etc. Establish good actions and inappropriate actions. The child with an otitis media history may not be able to change overnight, but does need to be made aware of more appropriate responses in interpersonal communication.
4.9.c Facilitate the child's language whenever possible, ie: expand his/her verbal skills through interaction.	**4.9.c.1** Facilitation is defined as "interacting with the child by following the child's lead in play and talking, using verbal techniques such as labelling, expansion, and parallel talking." (Hubbell, 1977) This strengthens the linguistic code. As the child's linguistic world is made easier, he/she can cope with other situations more easily.

Techniques for Curriculum Adaptation	Extra Information, Materials or References

4.9 The child is often unaware of the needs of others (also the intentions of others). (Continued)

4.9.c.2   For example: The child says: "My kitten bited and scratched me." The teacher resonse, "Oh, your kitten bit and scratched you." The child's ear hears the correction and in time, may correct the language himself/herself.

4.10 The child is often considered "immature."

4.10.a   Encourage more interactive play involving communication and social skills.

4.10.a.1   The child often appears to be "immature" in a variety of settings. Those settings usually are related to situations where the language task has become too complex or a situation where the child's self-esteem is at stake. For example, an otitis media affected child may react "immaturely" in a social situation where a verbal response is required. To put the child 'on the spot' verbally even if it's a simple response, may be too much for the child internally. The "immature" response may also become a learned response when the child is forced into that situation often. The child has to feel good enough about himself/herself, his/her linguistic capabilities and his/her audience before the child will respond maturely.

SOCIALIZATION

Techniques for Curriculum Adaptation	Extra Information, Materials or References

4.11 The child has difficulty taking turns.

4.11.a Praise the child when he/she allows another child to do something first.

4.11.a.1 The child is functioning in his/her own orderly world. Although the child has to function in the real world, until his/her linguistic structures make him/her more confident about himself/herself and the environment, he/she will not extend himself/herself. When the child begins to make the slightest headway, give praise such as "It was nice to see that you let Mary go first today." You've made reference to something which was a difficult task for the child. It may encourage him/her to try it again.

4.11.b Make allowances for the child's need to be first.

4.11.b.1 Because the child has difficulty taking turns, structure the situations so that turn taking is needed minimally. For example, if the crayons need to be shared, have enough for all. If two children want the same one, then establish class rules for sharing as you deem appropriate.

4.11.c Encourage more free play activity.

4.11.c.1 Start out with two children interacting, because three children often cause "splits" with the otitis media affected child left out.

Techniques for Curriculum Adaptation	Extra Information, Materials or References

4.12 The child can't wait to say what his/her thoughts are (also applies to the child who simply shouts out answers).

4.12.a Provide the child with opportunities to expand his/her immediate recall skills.

4.12 a.1 The child may have difficulty remembering things within a short time span. Internally, the child is aware of this and may want to express his/her ideas quickly before he/she forgets them. The child needs to communicate and feels badly when he/she forgets what he/she wants to say. The child needs to maintain a positive self-esteem.

4.12.b Provide a fairly quiet environment for communication interaction to cut down on external interference.

4.12 b.1 The child may be better able to retain his/her thought if extraneous interference such as noise or physical movement is kept at a minimum.

4.12.c Encourage the child by letting him/her know that you want to hear what he/she has to say and that you know it is important, but to wait for his/her turn to speak.

4.12 c.1 The child is often afraid that he/she may not have a chance to express the idea that took a while for him/her to formulate. As the child is often working with depressed linguistic skills, it takes a lot of work to put the thought together and the child feels that it's urgent to express it.

4.12.d Discuss communication and personal interaction skills with the whole class.

4.12 d.1 The child has been making sense to his/her world by looking out for himself/herself. This has kept his/her world orderly. The child often is unaware of the subtleties of inflection and stress patterns of people's speech and may therefore not be aware of the needs of others. He/she may not understand why he/she must wait to express his/her ideas at times

SOCIALIZATION

Techniques for Curriculum Adaptation	Extra Information, Materials or References

4.12 **The child can't wait to say what his/her thoughts are** (also applies to the child who simply shouts out answers). (Continued)

4.12 d.2 This may have to be discussed many times because the child may not be able to comprehend the topic on one try.

4.12 d.3 An organized system may have to be established through which the child becomes aware of the needs of others in classroom discussions. For example: have a special cue for the child such as an eye wink which can say to the child that you see his/her hand raised and will not forget to call on him, but try to wait patiently.

4.12 d.4 A trained response system of turn taking is easier in a small classroom. The fewer children in the classroom, the less time the child has to wait for his/her turn.

4.13 **The child prefers the company of younger children or adults.**

4.13.a Guide the child toward interactive play with one other child only.

4.13 a.1 This behavior demonstrates the way the child controls his/her auditory world to find social acceptance. The younger child probably more closely approximates his/her play level and linguistic level so that he/she is accepted. The adult is willing to accept what the child is doing, will interact and explain things to him and not have as many extraneous or busy movements to distract the child.

Techniques for Curriculum Adaptation	Extra Information, Materials or References

4.13   **The child prefers the company of younger children or adults. (Continued)**

4.13.b   Suggest small groups of two or four children for a group activity.

4.13.b1   A group of two or four members allows the children to be in pairs. A group of three children can sometimes isolate the one member that does not blend in as well.

Appendix A

BEHAVIORAL CHECKLIST

The following checklist of difficulties associated with the otitis media affected child in general has been helpful to the author as a basis for identifying a child at risk. It can be used either as a guideline for possible identification or as a screening tool. However, thorough assessment is necessary before you can make a definite diagnosis.

BEHAVIORAL CHECKLIST

Child's Name _____ Initial Intake Date _____ Second Intake Date _____

Classroom Teacher _____ Date of Birth _____ Age _____

Please check the following behaviors as they pertain to the child listed above.

	Initial Intake				Second Intake			
	Never	Seldom	Often	Other (Explain)	Never	Seldom	Often	Other (Explain)
1. Child seeks input from senses other than auditory (needs to physically touch others or to watch other's movements before attempting to follow through with task).								
2. Child uses vowel distortions in speech (EX: 'guwl' for 'girl').								
3. Child enjoys being read to.								
4. Child has difficulty attending to a listening task for a long period of time (not including being read to or watching TV).								
5. Child says 'huh?' or 'what?' frequently.								
6. Child functions best in orderly environment.								
7. Child prefers to play with one or two children versus a group.								
8. Child has difficulty recalling names of objects.								
9. Child has difficulty answering a simple question.								
10. Child has difficulty attending in the presence of background noise.								
11. Child is often unaware of the needs of others.								
12. Child may act out when situation is stressful (clings to mom, tantrums, crying, etc.).								
13. Child has difficulty following through with verbal directions.								
14. Child has delayed responses to sound.								
15. Child has difficulty waiting for turn.								
16. Child takes things very literally.								

from Davis, Dorinne. *Otitis Media: Coping with the Effects in the Classroom.* Hear You Are, Inc.: Stanhope, NJ, 1989.

Appendix B

The following Health Information Sheet can also be useful in identifying children who have had a significant history of Otitis Media. It will also help the children who were affected during their first two years of life and thus are also at risk for problems. This form can be given to all parents at the beginning of the school year and can serve as a part of an identification screening.

EAR HEALTH HISTORY

CHILD'S NAME _____ DOB _____ DATE _____

INFORMANT _____ CHILD'S AGE _____

Please help us better understand your child by answering the following questions:

1. Does your child have normal hearing (when ears are clear and healthy)?

   _____

2. Did your child ever have any ear infections?_____ If so, how many total?

   Between birth to 1 year old _____   3 to 4 years old _____

   1 to 2 years old_____   4 to 5 years old_____

   2 to 3 years old_____   5+ years _____

   How long did the ear infections last? _____

   How often did they re-occur? _____

3. Has your child had myrongotomies and PE tubes inserted?_____
   If so, how many times and at what ages?_____

4. Has your child received speech/language therapy?_____
   If so, at what ages and for how long?_____
   Therapy was for_____ articulation, _____
   language or other _____ (Please explain_____)

5. Has your child received amplification during periods of not hearing?

   _____

6. Is there anything else in your child}s ear health history that may be helpful in understanding your child's educational needs?_____

   _____
   _____

7. What concerns do you have about your child and school?_____

   _____
   _____

from Davis, Dorinne. *Otitis Media: Coping with the Effects in the Classroom.* Hear You Are, Inc.: Stanhope, NJ, 1989.

Appendix C

Sound Field Amplification

Audio Enhancement
932 Spoede Road North
St. Louis, MO 63146
1-314-567-6141

Hear You Are, Inc.
4 Musconetcong Avenue
Stanhope, NJ 07874
1-201-347-7662

Phonic Ear, Inc.
250 Camino Alto
Mill Valley, CA 94941
1-800-227-0735

Personal Sound Amplifiers

Audex
P.O. Box 3263
713 N. 4th Street
Longview, TX 75606
1-800-237-0716

Hear You Are, Inc.
4 Musconetcong Avenue
Stanhope, NJ 07874
1-201-347-7662

One to One
1714 Penrose
Olathe, KS 66062
1-813-764-4072

Telex
9600 Aldrich Avenue S.
Minneapolis, MN 55420
1-800-423-1559

Williams Sound Corp.
5929 Baker Road
Minnetonka, MN 55345-5997
1-612-931-0291

Sound Enhancement Systems

Audio Enhancement
932 Spoede Road North
St. Louis, MO 63146
1-314-567-6141

Hear You Are, Inc.
4 Musconetcong Avenue
Stanhope, NJ 07874
1-201-347-7662

Phonic Ear, Inc.
250 Camino Alto
Mill Valley, CA 94941
1-800-227-0735

Telex
9600 Aldrich Avenue S.
Minneapolis, MN 55420
1-800-423-1559

Periodicals

"Gifted Underachiever In Your Classroom?" *NEA Today*, Vol. 6, No. 9, April 1988, pp. 10 - 11.

"Hearing: A Link to IQ?" *Newsweek*, June 14, 1976, p. 97.

"Low Self-Esteem Often Leads to Student Failure." *NEA Today*, Vol. 7, No. 7, February 1989, p. 6.

"Middle Ear Fluid." *Parents' Pediatric Reports*, Report 20, April 1987.

"Middle Ear Infection." *The Harvard Medical School Health Letter*, Vol. VIII, No. 8, May 1982, pp. 1, 2 and 5.

"Screening Study Gives Clues on Children's Hearing Loss." *Hearing Instruments*, Vol. 34, No. 12, 1983, p. 23.

"We Can Give Kids An Edge On Survival." *NJEA Review*, February 1983, pp. 20 - 21.

Adelman, Howard S. "The Not So Specific Disability Population." *Exceptional Children*, Vol. 37, March 1971, pp. 528 - 533.

Allen, Doris V., and Robinson, Dale O. "Middle Ear Status and Language Development in Preschool Children" *ASHA*. June 1984, pp. 33 - 37.

Anderson, Karen L. "When 'Normal' Hearing is Not Normal." *Hear and Now*, Vol. 4, No. 4, March/April 1988, pp. 1 - 6.

Barton, P. T. "Auditory Disorders in Poor Readers." *Eyes, Ears, Nose and Throat Monthly*, Vol. 46, 1967, pp. 15 - 17.

Batin, R. *Corti's Organ*, Vol. 2, No. 3, 1977, pp. 2 - 3.

Bavosi, Robert P., and Rupp, Ralph R. "Otitis Media in Children - Further Findings on Spontaneous Resolution." *Hearing Journal*, February 1984, pp. 18.

Bavosi, Robert P., and Rupp, Ralph R. "When 'Normal' Hearing is not Normal." *Hearing Instruments*, Vol. 25, No. 9, 1984, pp. 9 and 39.

Bennett, Forrest C.; Ruuskea, Susan H.; and Sherman, Roberta. "Middle Ear Function in Learning-Disabled Children." *Pediatrics*, Vol. 66, No. 2, August 1980, pp. 254 - 259.

Beratis, S.; Rubin, M.; Miller, R. T.; Galenson, E.; and Rothstein, A. "Developmental Aspects of an Infant with Transient Moderate to Severe Hearing Impairment." *Pediatrics*, Vol. 1, 1979, pp. 153 - 155.

Berlin, L. F.; Blank, M.; and Rose, S. A. "The Language of Instruction: The Hidden Complexities." *Topics of Language Disorders*, Vol. 1, 1980, pp. 47 - 58.

Bluestone, Charles D.; Beery, Quinter; and Paradise, Jack L. "Audiometry and Tympanometry in Relation to Middle Ear Effusions in Children." *Laryngoscope*, Vol. 83, 1973, pp. 594 - 604.

Bluestone, Charles D.; Klein, Jerome O.; Paradise, Jack L.; Eichenwald, Heinz; Bess, Fred; Downs, Marion P.; Green, Morris; Berko-Gleason, Jean; Ventry, Ira M.; Gray, Susan W.; McWilliams, Jane; and Gates, George A. "Workshop on Effects of Otitis Media on the Child." *Pediatrics*, Vol. 71, No. 4, April 1983, pp. 639 - 652.

Brackett, Diane and Maxon, Antonia Brancia. "Service Delivery Alternatives for the Mainstreamed Hearing-Impaired Child." *American Speech-Language-Hearing Association*, Vol. 17, April 1986, pp. 115 - 125.

Brandes, Pauline, and Ehinger, Diane M. "Effects of Early Middle Ear Pathology on Auditory Perception and Academic Achievement." *Journal of Speech and Hearing Disorders*, Vol. 46, August 1981, pp. 301 - 307.

Brooks, Denzil N. "Otitis Media and Child Development." *Annals of Otology, Rhinology and Laryngology*, Vol. 88 , Suppl 60), No. 5, Pt. 2, September/October 1979, pp. 29 - 47.

Brown, William R. Jr. "Treating Ear Infections - Seriously and Immediately." *Mothers' Manual*. March/April 1981, pp. 14 and 17.

Burgener, Gerald W., and Mouw, John T. "Minimal Hearing Loss's Effect On Academic/Intellectual Performance of Children." *Hearing Instruments*, Vol. 33, No. 6, 1982, pp. 7 - 8 and 17.

Callazo, M. J., and Kricos, P. B. "Otitis-Prone Children and the Need for Speech/Language Services." *Hearing Instruments*, No. 37, 1986, pp. 14 - 19.

Camarata, Stephen, M.; Hughes, Charles, A.; and Ruhl, Kathy L. "Mild/Moderate Behaviorally Disordered Students: A Population at Risk for Language Disorders." *Language, Speech, and Hearing Services in Schools*, Vol. 19, April 1988, pp. 191-200.

Cantekin, Erdem I.; Mandel, Ellen; Bluestone, Charles D.; Rockette, Howard E.; Paradise, Jack L.; Stool, Sylvan E.; Fria, Thomas J.; and Rogers, Kenneth D. "Lack of Efficacy of a Decongestant-Antihistamine Combination for Otitis Media with Effusion ('Secretory Otitis Media) in Children." *The New England Journal of Medicine*, Vol. 308, No. 6, 1983, pp. *552 - 301*.

Cantwell, D. P., and Baher, L. "Psychiatric Disorder in Children with Speech and Language Retardation." *Archives of General Psychiatry*, Vol. 34, 1977, pp. 583 - 591.

Cantwell, Denis P., and Baker, Lorian. "Psychiatric and Behavioral Characteristics of Children with Communication Disorders." *Journal of Pediatric Psychology*, Vol. 5, No. 2, 1980, pp. 161 - 178.

Caplin, D. "A Special Report of Retardation of Children with Impaired Hearing in New York City Schools." *American Annals Deaf*, Vol. 82, 1937, pp. 234 - 243.

Cass, Richard, and Kaplan, Phyllis. "Middle Ear Disease and Learning Problems: A School System's Approach to Early Detection." *The Journal of School Health*. December 1979, pp. 557 - 560.

Casselbrant, Margareth L.; Brostoff, Leon M.; Cantekin, Erdem; Flaherty, Mildred; Doyle, William J.; Bluestone, Charles D.; and Fria, Thomas J. "Otitis Media with Effusion in Preschool Children." *Laryngoscope*, Vol. 95: April 1985, pp. 428 - 436.

Catts, Hugh W., and Kamhi, Alan G. "The Linguistic Basis of Reading Disorders: Implications for the Speech-Language Pathologist." *Language Speech and Hearing Services in Schools*, Vol. 17, October 1986, pp. 329 - 341.

Clark, John Greer. "The Hearing Aid Consultant and the Classroom Teacher." *Hearing Instrument*. Vol. 37, No. 9, 1986. p. 12.

Cohen, D., and Sade, J. "Hearing in Secretory Otitis Media." *Canadian Journal of Otolaryngology*, Vol. 1, No. 1, 1972, pp. 27 - 29.

Collazo, Mary J., and Kricos, Patricia B. "Otitis-Prone Children and Need for Speech/Language Service." *Hearing Instruments*, Vol. 37, No. 7, 1986, pp. 14 - 19.

Connor, Brian H. "Otitis Media in Children." *Australian Family Physician*, Vol. 11, No. 9, September 1982, pp. 671 - 678.

Cook, Roger A., and Teel, Robert W., Jr. "Negative Middle Ear Pressure and Language Development." *Clinical Pediatrics*, 18, 1979, pp. 296 - 297.

Crum, Michael A., and Matkin, Noel D. "Room Acoustics: The Forgotten Variable." *Language, Speech and Hearing Services in School*, Vol. VII, 1976, pp. 106 - 110.

Davis, Dorinne. "Kinnelon Schools Are First To Use Listenaider." Lakeland, NJ: *Lakeland Today*, January 17, 1988.

Davis, Dorinne. "Middle Ear Infections: Impact on Child." Hackensack, NJ: *The Record*, September 25, 1988, p. A47.

Davis, Dorinne. "Middle Ear Infections: The Social Impact." *Educational Audiology Newsletter*, Spring, 1988.

Davis, Robert, and Hamernik, Roger. "Does Otitis Media Cause Sensorineural Hearing Loss? An Overview." *The Hearing Journal*, Vol. 42, No. 3, March 1989.

Dobie, Robert A. and Berlin, Charles I. "Influence of Otitis Media on Hearing and Development." *Annals of Otology, Rhinology and Laryngology*, Vol. 88 (Supplement 60), 1979, pp. 48 - 53.

Dopheide, William R. and Dallinger, Jane R. "Preschool Articulation Screening by Parents." *Language Speech and Hearing Services in Schools*, VII, 1986, pp. 124 - 127.

Downs, Marion S., and Bergman, Florence B. "Otitis Prone Child." *Journal of Developmental and Behavioral Pediatrics*, Vol. 3, No. 2, June 1982, pp. 106 - 112.

Downs, Marion. "Effects of Mild Hearing Loss on Auditory Processing." *Otolaryngologic Clinics of North America*, Vol. 18, No. 2, May 1985, pp. 337 - 343.

Doyle, Janet. "Audiologists' Predictions of Speech Intelligibility from Pure-Tone Audiograms." *The Volta Review*, Vol. 90, No. 3, April 1988, pp. 155 - 164.

Eichenwald, Heinz. "Development in Diagnosing and Treating Otitis Media." *A.F.P.*, Vol. 31, No. 3, March 1985, pp. 155 - 163.

Eisen, Nathaniel Herman. "Some Effects of Early Sensory Deprivation On Later Behavior: The Quondam Hard-of-Hearing Child." *Journal of Abnormal and Social Psychology*, Vol. 65, No. 5, 1962, pp. 338 - 342.

Eliachar, Isaac. "Audiologic Manisfestations in Otitis Media." *Otolaryngologics Clinics of North America*, Vol. 11, No. 3, October 1978, pp. 769 - 776.

Elliott, Lois L., and Hammer, Michael A. "Longitudinal Changes in Auditory Discrimination in Normal Children with Language-Learning Problems." *Journal of Speech and Hearing Disorders*, Vol. 53, 1988, pp. 467 - 474.

Elssman, Sharon F.; Matkin, Noel D.; and Sabo, Michael P. "Early Identification of Congenital Sensorineural Hearing Impairment." *The Hearing Journal*, Vol. 40, No. 9, September 1987, pp. 13 - 17.

Fisch, L. "Otitis Media has a Deleterious Effect on...." *British Journal of Audiology*, Vol. 17, 1983, pp. 131 - 135.

Flavell, John H.; Beach, David R.; and Chinsky, Jack M. "Spontaneous Verbal Rehearsal in a Memory Task as a Function of Age." *Child Development*. June, 1966, pp. 283 - 299.

Flexer, Carol, and Ireland, JoAnne C. "Infant Otitis Media: A Case Study." *Hearing Instruments*, Vol. 37, No. 2, 1986, pp. 23 - 25, 50.

Freeman, Barry A., and Parkins, Charles. "The Prevalence of Middle Ear Disease Among Learning Impaired Children." *Clinical Pediatrics*, Vol. 18, No. 4 (April 1979). pp. 205 - 212.

Freeman, Barry A., and Parkins. "The Prevalence of Middle Ear Disease Among Learning Impaired Children." *Clinical Pediatrics*, Vol. 18, No. 4, April 1979, pp. 205 - 212.

Fria, Thomas J. *Corti's Organ*, Vol. 2, No. 3, 1977, pp. 1 - 2.

Fria, Thomas J.; Cantekin, Erdem I.; and Eichler, John A. "Hearing Acuity of Children with Otitis Media with Effusion." *Arch Otolaryngol*, Vol. III, January 1985, pp. 10 - 16.

Friel-Patti, Sandy; Finitzo, Terese; Myerhoff, William L.; and Hieber, J. Patrick. "Speech-Language Learning and Early Middle Ear Disease: A Procedural Report." *Otitis Media and Child Development*, J. Kavanagh (ed.) Parkton, MD: York Press, 1986.

Friel-Patti, Sandy; Finitzo-Nieber, Terese; Conti, Gina; and Brown, Karen Brown. "Language Delay in Infants Associated with Middle Ear Disease and Mild, Fluctuating Hearing Impairment." *Pediatric Infectious Disease*, Vol. 1, No. 2, 1982, pp. 104 - 109.

Gardner, Harvey J. "Moderate Vs. Colder Weather Effects on Hearing Screening, Results Among Preschool Children." *The Hearing Journal*, Vol. 4, No. 3, March 1988, pp. 29 - 32.

Gardner, Harvey J. "Application of a High Frequency Consonant. Discrimination Word List in Hearing-Aid Application." *Journal of Speech and Hearing Disorders*, Vol. 36, August 1971, pp. 354 - 355.

Garrard, Kay Russell, and Clark, Bertha Smith. "Otitis Media: The Role of Speech-Language Pathologists." *ASHA*. July 1985, pp. 35 - 38.

Gdowski, Becky; Sanger, Dixie D.; and Decker, T. Newell. "Otitis Media: Effect on a Child's Learning." *Academic Therapy*, Vol. 21, No. 3, January 1986, pp. 283 - 290.

Goetziner, C. P.; Harrison, Cliff; and Ball, C. J. "Small Perceptive Hearing Loss: Its Effect in School-Age Children." *The Volta Review*, Vol. 64, 1964, pp. 124 - 131.

Goetzinger, C. P., and Proud, G. O. "The Impact of Hearing Impairment Upon the Psychological Development of Children." *Journal of Auditory Research*, Vol. 15, 1975, pp. 1 - 60.

Goetzinger, C. P.; Harrison, C.; and Baer, C. J. "Small Perceptive Hearing Loss: Its Effect in School-Age Children." *The Volta Review*, Vol. 66, No. 3, 1964, pp. 124 - 131.

Goetzinger, Cornelius. "Effects of Small Perceptive Losses on Language and on Speech Discrimination." *The Volta Review*, Vol. 64, 1962, pp. 408 - 414.

Goinz, James B. "Otitis Media Among Pre-School and School Age Indian Children in MI, MN and WI." *Hearing Instruments*, Vol. 35, No. 6, 1984, pp. 16 and 18.

Goodhill, V., and Holcomb, A. "The Relation of Auditory Response to the Viscosity of Tympanic Fluids." *Acta Oto-Laryngologica*, Vol. 49, 1958, pp. 38 - 46.

Gottlieb, Marvin I.;Zinkus, Peter W.; and Thompson, Anne. "Chronic Middle Ear Disease and Auditory Perceptual Deficits." *Clinical Pediatrics*, Vol. 18, No. 12, December 1979, pp. 725 - 732.

Harris, Robert. "Central Auditory Functions in Children." *Perceptual and Motor Skills*, Vol. 16, 1963, pp. 207 - 214.

Harrison, Robert V., "The Physiology of Sensorineural Hearing Loss." *Hearing Instruments*. Vol. 37, No. 6, 1986, pp. 20, 22, 24, 26.

Harvey, Michael A. "Between Two Worlds: One Psychologist's View of the Hard of Hearing Person's Experience." *SHHH*, July/August, 1985, pp. 4 - 5.

Hasenstab, M. Suzanne, "Child Language Studies: Impact on Habilitation of Hearing-Impaired Infants and Preschool Children." *The Volta Review*, Vol. 85, 1983, pp. 88 - 100.

Hefferman, P. *Corti's Organ*, Vol. 2, No. 3, 1977, p. 4.

Hine, W. D. "The Attainments of Children with Partial Hearing." *Teacher of the Deaf*, Vol. 68, 1970, pp. 129 - 135.

Hodes, David S. "A Wolf in Sheep's Clothing: A Benign Bacterium Turns Pathogenic." *The Hearing Journal*, Vol. 40, No. 9, September 1987, pp. 31 - 32.

Hoffman - Lawless, Kimberly; Keith, Robert W.; and Cotton, Robin T. "Auditory Processing Abilities in Children with Previous Middle Ear Effusion." *Annals Otology*, Vol. 90, 1981, pp. 543 - 545.

Holm, Vanja, and Kunze, LuVern H. "Effect of Chronic Otitis Media on Language and Speech Development." *Pediatrics*, Vol. 43, No. 5, May 1969, pp. 833 - 830.

Houchins, R.; Pearson, M.; and Carson, P. "An Inservice Training Program to Assist Regular Classroom Teachers in Serving the Mildly Hearing Impaired." *Journal of the ARA*, Vol. XII, No. 2, 1979, pp. 86 - 94.

Howie, Virgil M. "The 'Otitis-Prone' Condition," *American Journal Disordered Children*, Vol. 129, 1975, p. 676.

Howie, Virgil M. "Developmental Sequelae of Chronic Otitis Media, a Review." *Journal of Developmental and Behavioral Pediatrics*, Vol. 1, No. 1, March 1980, pp. 34 - 38.

Howie, Virgil M.; Jensen, Norma J.; Fleming, James W.; Peeler, Milton B.; and Meigs, Stanley. "The Effect of Early Onset of Otitis Media on Education Achievement." *International Journal of Pediatric Otorhinlaryngology*, Vol. 1, 1979, pp. 151 - 155.

Howie, Virgil M.; Ploussard, John H.; and Sloyer, John. 'The "Otitis-Prone" Condition.' *American Journal of Dis. Child*, Vol. 129, June 1975, pp. 676 - 678.

Ickes, William K., and Keel, Dale. "High Prevalence of Otitis Media Among Indian Children: Fact or Myth." *Hearing Instruments*, Vol. 33, No. 2, 1982, pp. 22 - 24, 63.

Imgley, S. P., and Thomure, F. E. "Some Effects of Hearing Impairments Upon School Performance." *Division of Special Education Services*, Office of the Supt. of Public Instruction, State of Illinois, 1970.

Ireland, JoAnn; Flexer, Carol; and Wray, Denise. "Preferential Seating is Not Enough: Issues in Classroom Management of Hearing-Impaired Students." *Language, Speech and Hearing Services in Schools*, Vol. 20, Jan 1989, pp. 11 - 21.

Jerger, Susan; Jerger, James; Alford, Bobby R.; and Abrams, Sue. "Development of Speech Intelligibility in Children with Recurrent Otitis Media." *Ear and Hearing*, Vol. 4, No. 3, 1983, pp. 138 - 145.

Kantrowitz, Barbara, and Wingert, Pat. "How Kids Learn." *Newsweek*, April 17, 1989, pp. 50 - 56.

Kaplan, Gary J.; Fleshman, J. Kenneth; Bender, Thomas R.; Baum, Carol; and Clark, Paul S. "Long Term Effects of Otitis Media, A Ten Year Cohort Study of Alaskan Eskimo Children." *Pediatrics*, Vol. 52, No. 4, October 1973, pp. 577 - 584.

Katz, Jack, and Burge, Cena. "Auditory Perception Training for Children With Learning Disabilities." *Menorah Medical Journal*, Vol. 2, 1971, pp. 18 - 29.

Katz, Jack. "Temporary Threshold Shift, Auditory Sensory Deprivation, and Conductive Hearing Loss." *Journal Acoustical Society of America*, Vol. 37, 1965, pp. 293 - 294.

Katz, Jack. "The Effects of Conductive Hearing Loss on Auditory Function." *ASHA*, Vol. 20, October 1978, pp. 879 - 885.

Kessler, Maurine E., and Randolph, Kenneth. "The Effects of Early Middle Ear Disease on the Auditory Abilities of Third Grade Children." *Journal of Academic Rehabilitative Audiology*, Vol. 12, No. 2, October 1979, pp. 6 - 20.

Kile, Jack E., and Lauten, Mary F. "The Application of an Auditory Training Method." *Hearing Instruments*, Vol. 9, No. 9, 1986, pp. 35, 36 and 63.

Köhler, Lënnart, and Holst, Hans-Eric. "Auditory Screening of Four-Year-Old Children." *Acta Paediat Scandinavia*, Vol. 6, 1967, pp. 555 - 560.

Köhler, Lënnart, and Holst, Hans-Eric. "Auditory Screening of Four-Year-Old Children." *Acta Paediat Scandinavia*, Vol. 61, 1972, pp. 555 - 560.

Kreimeyer, Kathryn, and Anita, Skirin. "The Development and Generalization of Social Interaction Skills in Preschool Hearing-Impaired Children." *The Volta Review*, May 1988, pp. 219 - 239.

LaCoste, Mary. "School Learning Problems - Are Chronic Ear Infections in the Preschool Years a Cause?" *Speaking of Hearing*, Spring 1984, pp. 5 - 6.

Lambert, Frances; Ericksen, Nancy; Blickham, Janice; and Hollister, Sharon. "Listening and Language Activities for Preschool Children." *Language, Speech and Hearing Services in School*, Vol. XI, April 1980, pp. 111 - 117.

Lehmann, M. Drue; Charron, Kathy; Kummer, Ann; and Keith, Robert W. "The Effects of Chronic Ear Effusion on Speech and Language Development - A Descriptive Study." *International Journal of Pediatric Otorhinolaryngology*, Vol. 1, 1979, pp. 137 - 144.

Leviton, Alan. "Otitis Media and Learning Disorders." *Developmental and Behavioral Pediatrics*, Vol. 1, No. 2, June 1980, pp. 58 - 62.

Lewis, Neil. "Otitis Media and Linguistic Incompetence." *Arch Otolarynol*, Vol. 102, July 1976, pp. 387 - 390.

Ling, Agnes. "Training of Auditory Memory in Hearing Impaired Children: Some Problems of Generalization." *Journal of the American Audiology Society*, Vol. 1, No. 4, 1976, pp. 150 - 157.

Longhurst, T., and Siegel, G. "Effects of Communication Failure on Speaker and Listener Behavior." *Journal of Speech and Hearing Research*, Vol. 16, 1973, pp. 128 - 140.

Lovas, Dorinne. "Pre-School Sound Field Amplification." *The Directive Teacher*, Vol. 9, No. 1, Summer/Fall 1986, pp. 22 - 23.

Luria, A. R. "The Functional Organization of the Brain." *Scientific American*. March 1970, pp. 66 - 78.

Mahon, William. "Hearing Care for Infants and Children." *The Hearing Journal*, September 1987, pp. 7 - 11.

Mandel, Ellen M.; Rackette, Howard E.; Bluestone, Charles D; Paradise, Jack L.; and Nozza, Robert J. "Efficacy of Amoxicilian With and Without Decongestant Antihistamine for Otitis Media with Effusion in Children." *The New England Journal of Medicine*, Vol. 316, No. 8, Feb. 19, 1987, pp. 432 - 437.

Marston, L. E., and Larkin, Maureen. "Auditory Assessment of Reading Underachieving Children." *Language, Speech and Hearing Services in Schools*, Vol. X, October 1979, pp. 212 - 230.

Master, Lowell, and Marsh, George E. "Middle Ear Pathology as a Factor in Learning Disabilities." *Journal of Learning Disabilities*, Vol. 11, No. 2, 1978, pp. 54 - 57.

Matkin, N. *Corti's Organ*, Vol. 2, No. 3, 1977, p. 3.

McDaniel, Mark, and Kearney, Edmund. "Optimal Learning Strategies and Their Spontaneous Use: The Importance of Task-Appropriate Processing." *Memory and Cognition*, Vol. 12, No. 4, 1984, pp. 361 - 373.

McGee, R.; Silva, P. A.; and Stewart, I. A. "Behavior Problems and Otitis Media with Effusion: A Report from the Dunedin Multidisciplinary Child Development Study." *New Zealand Medical Journal*, Vol. 95, 1982, pp. 655 - 657.

McKerrow, Kelly. "The Educational Effects of Mild Hearing Loss and Middle Ear Pressure." *Hearing Instruments*, Vol. 39, No. 9. 1988, pp. 34, 36, 38.

McLaughlin, Loretta. "Infant Ear Disease Difficult to Detect." *Boston Sunday Globe*, May 16, 1976.

McLaughlin, Loretta. "Minor Hearing Loss Becoming Major Problem." *Boston Sunday Globe*, May 9, 1976, p. A20.

Mehta, Dinesh, and Erlich, Mark. "Serous Otitis Media in a School for the Deaf." *The Volta Review*, Vol. 80, No. 2, February/-March 1978, pp. 75-80.

Menyuk, Paula. "Design Factors in the Assessment of Language Development in Children with Otitis Media." *The Annals of Otology, Rhinology and Laryngology*, Vol. 88 (Supplement 60) No. 5 Pt. 2, September/October 1979, p 78 - 87.

Menyuk, Paula. "Syntactic Rules Used by Children from Preschool Through First Grade." *Child Development*, Vol. 35, 1964, pp. 533 - 546.

Miller, M. *Corti's Organ*, Vol. 2, No. 3, 1977, pp. 3 - 4.

Mira, Mary. "Individual Patterns of Looking and Listening Preferences Among Learning Disabled and Normal Children." *Exceptional Children*, May 1968, pp. 649 - 658.

Moore, Dorothy, and Best, Gilbert. "A Sensorineural Component in Chronic Otitis Media." *The Laryngoscope*, Vol. 90, 1980, pp. 1360 - 1365.

Mustain, William D. "Linguistic and Educational Implications of Recurrent Otitis Media." *Ear, Nose and Throat Journal*, Vol. 58, May 1979, pp. 62 - 67.

Naremore, Rita C. "Influence of Hearing Impairment on Early Language Development." *The Annals of Otology, Rhinology and Laryngology*, Vol. 88, (Supplement 60), No. 5 Pt. 2, September/October 1979, pp. 54 - 63.

Needleman, Harriet. "Effects of Hearing Loss From Early Recurrent Otitis Media on Speech and Language Development," in Jaffe, B. (ed.) *Hearing Loss in Children: A Comprehensive Text*. Baltimore, MD: University Park Press, 1977, pp. 640 - 649.

Olmsted, Richard W.; Alvarez, Milton C.; Moroney, John D.; and Eversden, Marguerite. "The Pattern of Hearing Following Acute Otitis Media." *The Journal of Pediatrics*, Vol. 65, No. 2, August 1964, pp. 252 - 255.

Orloskie, Arthur J., and Leddo, John S. "Environmental Effects on Children's Hearing." *Journal of School Health*, January 1981, pp. 12 - 14.

Paradise, Jack L. "Otitis Media During Early Life: How Hazardous to Development? A Critical Review of the Evidence." *Pediatrics*, Vol. 68, 1981, pp. 869 - 871.

Paradise, Jack L. "Otitis Media in Infants and Children." *Pediatrics*, Vol. 65, No. 5, 1980, pp. 917 - 943.

Parmiter-Jacobs, Linda; Kraemer, Karen Black; and Jared, Carol. "When a Hearing Instrument is Not Enough: An ALD Center." *Hearing Instruments*, Vol. 39, No. 6, 1988, pp. 22 - 23.

Pearson, P. David, and Fielding, Linda. "Research Update: Listening Comprehension." *Language Arts*, Vol. 59, September 1982. pp. 617 - 629.

Peckham, Catherine; Sheridan, Mary; and Butler, Neville R. "School Attainment of Seven-Year-Old Children with Hearing Difficulties." *Developmental Medicine and Child Neurology*, Vol. 15, 1972, pp. 592 - 602.

Phelps, Diana. "A Modified Association Method: Remediation for L.D. Children." *Ohio Journal of Speech and Hearing*, Vol. 13, No. 2, Spring, 1978, pp. 93 - 104.

Pollack, Doreen. "The Crucial Year: A Time to Listen." *International Audiology*, Vol. 6, No. 2, 1967, pp. 243 - 247.

Quigley, S. P.; Power, D. J.; and Steinkamp, M. W. "The Language Structure of Deaf Children." *The Volta Review*, Vol. 79, February/March, 1977, pp. 73 - 84.

Radcliffe, Donald. "Rx for Otitis Media in Children." *The Hearing Journal*, Vol. 36, No. 16, June 1983, p. 14.

Ralabate, Patti, "What Teachers Should Know About Middle Ear Dysfunction." *NEA Today*, May 1987, p. 10.

Ralph, J. Clyde. "Hearing Loss, Learning Deficit." *Speaking of Hearing*, Fall 1984.

Rapin, Isabelle. "Conductive Hearing Loss Effects On Children's Language and Scholastic Skills." *Annals of Otology, Rhinology and Laryngology*, Vol. 88, 1979, pp. 3 - 12.

Ray, Helen; Sarff, Lewis; and Glassford, F. E. "Sound Field Amplification: An Innovative Educational Intervention for Mainstreamed Learning Disabled Students." *The Directive Teacher*, Vol. 6, No. 2, Summer/Fall 1984, pp. 18 - 20.

Reichman, Julie, and Healey, William C. "Learning Disabilities and Conductive Hearing Loss Involving Otitis Media." *Journal of Learning Disabilities*, Vol. 16, No. 5, (May 1983, pp. 272 - 278.

Rentschler, Gary J., and Rupp, Ralph R. "Conductive Hearing Loss: Cause for Concern?" *Hearing Instruments*, Vol. 35, No. 6, 1984, pp. 12 - 14.

Robarts, John T. "Impedance Screening - A Way to Prevent Learning Problems." *The Hearing Aid Journal*, May, 1979.

Robarts, John T. "Impedance in School Screening Programs." *Hearing Instruments*, Vol. 35, No. 2, 1983. pp. 8 - 11.

Roberts, Joanne Erwick; Burchinal, Margaret R.; Koch, Matthew A.; Footo, Marianna M.; and Henderson, Frederick W. "Otitis Media In Early Childhood and Its Relationship to Later Phonological Development." *American Speech-Language-Hearing Association*, Vol. 53, November 1988, pp. 424 - 432.

Robinson, Geoffrey; Anderson, Donald O.; Moghadam, Hossein K.; Cambon, Kenneth G.; and Murray, Andrew B. "A Survey of Hearing Loss in Vancouver School Children." *Canadian Medical Association Journal*, Vol. 97, November 1967, pp. 1199 - 1207.

Rose, Deborah; Lang, Janna Smith; and Fargo, Jennifer. "The Role of Hearing in Child Development: Rationale for Intervention." *Hearing Instruments*, Vol. 34, No. 10, 1983. pp. 22 - 31, 55.

Ross, Dorothea M., and Ross, Sheila A. "The Efficacy of Listening Training for Educable Mentally Retarded Children." *American Journal of Mental Deficiency*, Vol. 77, No. 2, 1972, pp. 137 - 142.

Ross, Mark, and Grolas, Thomas. "Effect of Three Classroom Listening Conditions on Speech Intelligibility." *A.A.D*, December 1971, pp. 580 - 584.

Ruben, R., and Rapin, J. "Plasticity of the Developing Auditory System." *Annals of Otolaryngology*, Vol. 89, 1980, pp. 303 - 311.

Ruben, Robert J. "Serous Otitis Media." *The Volta Review*, Vol. 80, No. 2, February/March 1978, pp. 73-74.

Ruben, Robert J., and Hanson, David G. "Summary of Discussion and Recommendation Made During the Workshop on Otitis Media and Development." *Annals of Otology, Rhinology and Laryngology*, Vol. 88, No. 5, Pt. 2, 1979, pp. 107-111.

Rubin, Martha. "Serious Otitis Media in Severely to Profoundly Hearing-Impaired Children, Ages 0 to 6." *The Volta Review*, Vol. 80, No. 2, February/March 1978, pp. 81 - 85.

Rupp, Ralph R. "A Review of the Auditory Processing Skills of Fifty Children and Recommendation for Educational Management." *Journal of the ARA*, Vol. XII, No. 2, 1979, pp. 63 - 85.

Rupp, Ralph R.; Jackson, Patricia D.; and McGill, Norma. "Listening Problems = Academic Distress." *Hearing Instruments*, Vol. 37, No. 9, 1986, pp. 20, 22, 24.

Rupp, Ralph R.; Steen, Kendra; and Babosi, Robert. "Conductive Hearing Losses: Subjective Reactions." *Hearing Instruments*, Vol. 38, No. 9, 1987, pp. 38, 40.

Sak, Robert J., and Ruben, Robert J. "Effects of Recurrent Middle Ear Effusion in Preschool Years on Language Learning." *Journal of Developmental and Behavioral Pediatrics*, Vol. 3, No. 1, March 1982, pp. 7 - 11.

Sanders, Derek. "Noise Conditions in Normal School Classrooms." *Exceptional Children*, March 1965, pp. *344 - 552*.

Sanger, Dixie D.; Freed, J. M.; and Decker, T. N. "Behavioral Profile of Pre-School Children 'At Risk' for Auditory-Language Processing Problems." *Hearing Journal*, Vol. 38, No. 10, 1985, pp. 17 - 20.

Sanger, Dixie D.; Keith, Robert W.; and Maher, Barbara Anne. "An Assessment Technique for Children with Auditory-Language Processing Problems." *Journal of Communication Disorders*, Vol. 20, No. 4, 1987, pp. 265 - 277.

Sarff, Lewis; Ray, Helen; and Bagwell, Cynthia. "Why Not Amplification in Every Classroom?" *The Hearing Journal*, Vol. 24, No. 10, October 1981.

Seltz, A. *Corti's Organ*, Vol. 2, No. 3, 1977, p. 1.

Senturia, Ben H.; Bluestone, Charles D; Klein, Jerome O.; Lim, David J.; and Paradise, Jack L. "Report of the Ad Hoc Committee on Definition and Classification of Otitis Media and Otitis Media with Effusion." *The Annals of Otology, Rhinology and Laryngology*, Vol. 89 (Suppl. 68), No. 3 Pt. 2, 1980, pp. 3 - 4.

Shah, C. P.; Chandler, D.; and Dale, R. "Delay in Referral of Children with Impaired Hearing". *The Volta Review*, Vol. 80, No. 4, May 1978, pp. 206 - 215.

Shapiro, Alvin, and Mistal, Gregory. "ITE-Aid Auditory Training for Reading and Spelling-Disabled Children: Clinical Case Studies." *The Hearing Journal*, Vol. 38, No. 3, February 1985, pp. 26 - 31.

Shirberg, Lawrence D. and Smith, Anne J. "Phonological Correlates of Middle-Ear Involvement in Speech-Delayed Children: A Methodological Note." *American Speech-Language-Hearing Association*, Vol. 26, June 1983, pp. 293 - 297.

Shoop, Mary. "Inquest: A Listening and Reading Comprehension Strategy." *The Reading Teacher*, Vol. 39, March 1986, pp. 670 - 674.

Shribert, Lawrence D., and Smith, Ann J. "Phonological Correlates of Middle-Ear Involvement in Speech-Delayed Children: A Methodological Note." *Journal of Speech and Hearing Research*, Vol. 26, June 1983, pp. 293 - 297.

Silva, Phil A.; Kirkland, Coralie; Simpson, Anne; Stewart, Ian A.; and Williams, Sheila. "Some Developmental and Behavioral Problems Associated with Bilateral Otitis Media with Effusion." *Journal of Learning Disabilities*, Vol. 15, No. 7, 1982, pp. 417 - 421.

Simmons, Audrey Ann. "Teaching Aural Language." *The Volta Review*, Vol. 70, No. 1, January 1968, pp. 26 - 30.

Skinner, Margaret Walker. "The Hearing of Speech During Language Acquisition." *Otolaryngolgic Clinics of North America*, Vol. 11, No. 3, October 197, pp. 631 - 650.

Smyth, Veronica. "Speech Reception in the Presence of Classroom Noise." *Language, Speech and Hearing Services in Schools*, Vol. X, October 1979, pp. 221 - 230.

Sprunt, Julie W., and Finger, Frank W. "Auditory Deficiency and Academic Achievement." *The Journal of Speech and Hearing Disorders*, Vol. 14, 1949, pp. 26 - 32.

Stubblefield, James H. "Longitudinal Study of Early Intervention in Middle Ear Dysfunction." *Hearing Instruments*, Vol. 33, No. 6, 1982, pp. 18 - 19 and 46.

Sudler, William H., and Flexer, Carol. "Low Cost Assistive Listening Device." *Language, Speech and Hearing Services in Schools*, Vol. 17, October 1986, pp. 342 - 344.

Teele, D. W., and Downs, M. "The High Risk Factors for Recurrent Otitis Media." *Annals of Otology*, Supplement 68, 1989, pp. 1 - 362.

Thomas, Ron. "A Curriculum Guide for Children With Chronic Middle Ear Problems." *Speaking of Hearing*, W. Newton, MA: Fall 1983.

Tobey, Emily; Cullen, John Jr.; Rampp, Donald; and Fleischer-Gallagher, Ann. "Effects of Stimulus-Onset Asynchrony on the Dichotic Performance of Children with Auditory-Processing Disorders." *Journal of Speech and Hearing Research*, Vol. 22, No. 2, June 1979, pp. 197 - 211.

Wallace, Ina F.; Gravel, Judith S.; McCarton, Cecelia M.; and Ruben, Robert J. "Otitis Media and Language Development at 1 year of Age." *Journal of Speech and Hearing Disorders*, Vol. 52, August 1988, pp. 245 - 251.

Weber, Harold J.; McGovern, Frank J.; and Zink, David. "An Evaluation of 1000 Children with Hearing Loss." *Journal of Speech and Hearing Disorders*, Vol. 32, 1967, pp. 343 - 354.

Webster, Douglas B., and Webster, Molly. "Effects of Neonatal Conductive Hearing Loss on Brain Stem Auditory Nuclei," *Annals of Otology, Rhinology and Laryngology*, Vol. 88, 1979, pp. 684 - 688.

Webster, Douglas B., and Webster, Molly. "Neonatal Sound Deprivation Affects Brain Stem Auditory Nuclei." *Arch. Otolaryngot*, Vol. 103, 1988, pp. 392 - 396.

Webster, Douglas, and Webster, Molly. "Mouse Brainstem Auditory Nuclei Development." *Annals of Otology, Rhinology and Laryngology*, Vol. 89 (Supplement 68), Pt. 2, May/June 1980, pp. 254 - 256.

Weiner, Lyn Ausberger. "Discovering Otitis Media: Diary of a Speech Pathologist." *The Directive Teacher*, Summer/Fall 1984, pp. 22 - 23.

White, Burton L. "The Critical Importance of Hearing Ability, Part 1." *Newsletter*, Vol. 1, No. 3, April 1979, pp. 1 - 3.

White, Burton L. "The Critical Importance of Hearing Ability, Part 2." *Newsletter*, Vol. 1, No. 4, June 1979, pp. 1 - 3.

Wiederhold, M. L.; Zajtchuk, J. T.; Vap, J. G.; and Paggi, R. E. "Hearing Loss in Relation to Physical Properties of Middle Ear Effusions." *The Annals of Otology, Rhinology and Laryngology*, Vol. 89 (Supplement 68), 1980, pp. 185 - 189.

Wilt, Miriam. "A Study of Teacher Awareness of Listening as a Factor in Elementary Education." *Journal of Educational Research*, Vol. 43, April 1950, pp. 626 - 636.

Windham, Robert. "The Auditory Processing of L.D. Children." *Hearing Instruments*, Vol. 36, No. 9, 1985, pp. 30 - 38.

Young, Patrick. "Middle Ear Infection Foiled if Caught Early." *Star Ledger*, April 26, 1987, p. 7.

Zinkus, Peter W., and Gottlieb, Marvin I. "Chronic Otitis Media and Auditory Processing Deficits: A Preventable Learning Disability." *Ohio Journal of Speech and Hearing*, Vol. 13, No. 2, Spring 1978, pp. 86 - 92.

Zinkus, Peter W., and Gottlieb, Marvin, I. "Patterns of Perceptual and Academic Deficits Related to Early Chronic Otitis Media." *Pediatrics*, Vol. 66, No. 2, August, 1980, pp. 246 - 252.

Zinkus, Peter W.; Gottlieb, Marvin I.; and Schapiro, Mark. "Developmental and Psychoeducational Sequelae of Chronic Otitis Media." *American Journal Disordered Children*, Vol. 132, November 1978, pp. 1100 - 1104.

Books

Berg, Frederick. *Educational Audiology Resource*. (Smithfield, VT: Ear Products & Services, 1985).

Berg, Frederick. *Educational Audiology: Hearing and Speech Management*. (New York: Grune & Stratton, Inc., 1976).

Berg, Frederick. *Facilitating Classroom Listening: A Handbook for Teachers of Normal and Hard of Hearing Students*. (Boston, MA: Little, Brown and Company, 1987).

Berg, Fredericks S.; Blair, James; Blair, C.; Viekweg, Steven H.; and Wilson-Vlotman, Ann. *Educational Audiology for the Hard of Hearing Child*. (Orlando, FL: Grune & Stratton, Inc., 1986).

Brierley, John. *Give Me A Child Until He Is Seven*. (Philadelphia, PA: The Falmer Press, 1988).

Brown, Sam. *What's That I Hear*. (Tucson, AZ: Communication Skill Builders, Inc., 1986).

Delfosse, Anne. *Auditory Processing in Action*. (Moline, IL: Lingui Systems, Inc., 1984).

Gillet, Pamela. *Auditory Processes*. (Novato, CA: Academic Therapy Publication, 1974).

Hasenstab, M. Suzanne. *Language Learning and Otitis Media*. (Boston, MA: College-Hill Press, 1987).

James, Muriel, and Jongeward, Dorothy. *Born to Win*. (New York: New American Library, 1978.)

Johnson, R.; Campbell, R.; and Mueller, P. *Improving Your Child's Listening and Language Skills: A Parent's Guide to Language Development*. (Toledo: Toledo Public Schools, October 1982).

Johnson, Ruth Ann. *Learning to Communicate Early in Life*. (Danville, IL: The Interstate Printers & Publishers, Inc., 1985).

Kavanagh, James F. *Otitis Media and Child Development*. (Parkton, MD: York Press, 1986).

Lindstrom, Deborah; Heron, Nancy; Polk, Christine; and Roach, Jane. *Comprehension Strategies and Activities*. (CIRP, Inc. 1976).

Lindstrom, Deborah; Polk, Christine; Roach, Jane; and Heron, Nancy. *Listening and Following Directions*. (CIRP, Inc. 1976).

Northern, J., and Downs, M. *Hearing in Children*. (Baltimore, MD: Williams & Wilkins, 1984).

Payne, Elizabeth E., and Paparella, Michael M. "Otitis Media." in J. Northern (ed) *Hearing Disorders*. (Boston: Little, Brown and Company, 1976).

Rampp, Donald L. *Classroom Activities for Auditory Perceptual Disorder*. (Danville, IL: The Interstate Printers & Publishers, Inc., 1976).

Ross, Mark. "Classroom Acoustics and Speech Intelligibility." in J. Katz (ed.) *Handbook of Clinical Audiology*, (Baltimore: Williams & Wilkins Co., 1972).

Tarnapol, Ed. "The Neurology of Learning Disabilities." in *Learning Disorders in Children: Diagnosis, Medication, and Education*. (Boston: Little, Brown & Co., 1971).

Vissher, Wendy H.; Mandel, Jack S.; Batalden, Paul B.; Russ, Joyce N,; and Giebink, Scott. "A Case-Control Study Exploring Possible Risk Factors for Childhood Otitis Media." in D. Lum, C. Bluestone, J. Klein and J. Nelson (Eds.), "Recent Advances in Otitis Media with Effusion." (Philadelphia: B.C. Decker, 1984).

Others Sources

"How to Foster Language Development." *The Hidden Handicap, Project C.H.I.L.D.* Toledo Public Schools, 1982.

"Low Level Amplification in the Classroom." *Teachers' Reactions on the System's Effectiveness*, Title IV-C, ESEA Project. Norris City, IL, 1977.

"Middle Ear Disease in Infancy: Current Concepts in Diagnosis and Management." Workshop in Cambridge, MA, March 16, 1985, by Boston University School of Medicine.

Barsky, Lisa. "Suggestions for Working With Children Who Exhibit Central Auditory Processing Deficits." March 23, 1984, Personal Contact.

Cazden, Courtney. "Two Paradoxes in the Acquisition of Language Structure and Functions." Paper presented at conference on the Development of Competence in Early Childhood. London, January 1972.

Cherry, Rochelle. "Development of Listening in Normal Achieving and Learning Disabled Children." Paper presented at NJSHA Convention, May 1980.

Churchill, Janine; Hodson, Barbara; Jones, Barry; and Noval, Robert. "Phonological Systems of Clients with Histories of Recurrent Otitis Media." Paper presented at ASHA Convention, Washington, DC, November 1985.

DeFrank, Lois Y. "Listening Skills Workshop." Lincoln School, January 25, 1972.

Downs, Marion. "Central Correlates of Hearing Loss." Presentation Notes, May 1984. New Brunswick, NJ.

Downs, Marion. "Otitis Media and Its Effect on Learning." One Day Workshop. Parsippany, NJ, April 4, 1984.

Downs, Marion. "The Upper Limits of Peripheral Loss. The Lower Limit of Hearing." Paper presented at NJSHA Convention. New Brunswick, NJ, 1984.

Edwards, Carolyn. "Seminar In Educational Audiology." Workshop Notes, August 4 - 8, 1988. Mississauga, Ontario, Canada.

Fischer, R., and Fitzgerald, M. D. "Identification and Management of Speech and Language Problems in Mild Hearing Loss." Paper presented at conference: The Problems of Children with Very Mild Hearing Loss: A Closer Look. Vanderbilt University, Nashville, TN, September 1982.

Friel-Patti, Sandy, and Finitzo, Terese. "Speech-Language Learning and Early Middle Ear Disease: Research Issues." Paper presented at American Speech-Language-Hearing Association Convention, Detroit, MI, November 1986.

Friel-Patti, Sandy; Finitzo, Terese; and Heiber, J. Patrick. "Communication Disorders Screening in a Pediatric Practice." Paper presented at the National Symposium on Hearing in Infants. Denver, CO, September 25, 1986.

Glassford, F. F.; Sorff, Lewis; and Ray, Helen. "Project M.A.R.R.S." Wabash and Ohio Valley Special Education District, Norris City, IL, 1977.

Goode, Richard. "What They Never Taught You About Middle Ear Pathology." Paper presented at ASHA Convention, New Orleans, LA, 1987.

Kersher, Evan, and Stern, Carolyn. "The Value of Spoken Response in Teaching Listening Skills to Young Children Through Programming Instruction." ED027 973. Washington, D.C. ERIC Document Reproduction Services, 1979.

Kinsbury, H. F., and Strumpf, F. M. "The Development and Testing of Guidelines for Designing School Classrooms to Maximize Hearing Conditions and Provide for Effective Noise Control." November 1969. ERIC Doc.: ED040 603.

Nozza, Robert J.; Carrigan, Victoria A.; Otte, Barbara; Bluestone, Charles D.; and Mandel, Ellen M. "Recent Findings from the Otitis Media Research Center." Children's Hospital of Pittsburgh, Miniseminar presented at the Annual Convention of the American Speech-Language-Hearing Association, New Orleans, LA, November 13 - 16, 1987.

Paden, Elane; Novak, Michael; and Kuklinski, Anne. "Otitis Media and Phonological Delay: An Avoidable Relationship." Paper presented at ASHA Convention, Washington, DC, November 1985.

Sanger, Dixie D.; Keith, Robert W.; Maher, Barbara A.; and Rusksdashel, Sharon V. "Intervention in Children with Auditory Processing Disorders." Presentation at American Speech-Language-Hearing Association Convention, November 1987.

Shrilberg, Lawrence D. "The Relation of Acoustic Constraints Associated with Otitis Media to Speech Perception and Production." Paper presented at American Speech-Language-Hearing Association Annual Convention, Detroit, MI, November 1986.

Taylor, Stanford. *Listening*, publ. by National Education Association of the United States, 1973.

Thulke, Helen, and Shriberg, Lawrence D. "Speech-Language Sequelae of Recurrent Otitis Media in Native American Preschoolers." Paper presented at the American Speech-Language-Hearing Association Convention, New Orleans, LA, November 1987.

Urban, Montgomery. "Educational Environment Modification for Students with Central Auditory Processing Problems." Montgomery Health Department. Silver Springs, MD, pp. 1 - 14.

Wesenger, Grace. *Awareness Workshop*. Regional Resource Center for Hearing Impairment. (Milton, QB, Canada: E.C. Drury), 1988.

White, Burton L. "Can Your Child Hear Well Enough to Learn?" (Philadelphia, PA: Scott Paper Company, 1980), pp. 1 - 5.